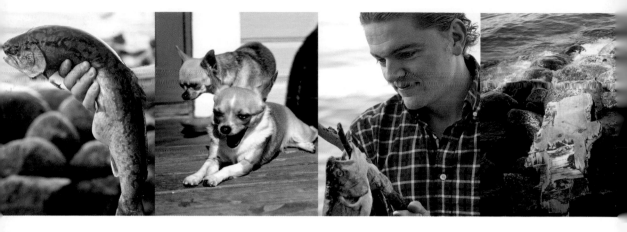

Skyhorse Publishing books may be purchased in bulk at special discounts for sales promotion, corporate gifts, fund-raising, or educational purposes. Special editions can also be created to specifications. For details, contact the Special Sales Department, Skyhorse Publishing,
307 West 36th Street, 11th Floor, New York, NY 10018 or info@skyhorsepublishing.com.

Skyhorse® and Skyhorse Publishing® are registered trademarks of Skyhorse Publishing, Inc.®,
a Delaware corporation.

www.skyhorsepublishing.com

10 9 8 7 6 5 4 3 2 1

Library of Congress Cataloging-in-Publication Data
Paulún, Fredrik, 1970-
  [LCHQ. English]
  Low carb, high quality diet : food for a thinner, healthier life / Fredrik Paulun ; translated by Viktoria Lindback.
     pages cm
  Includes bibliographical references and index.
  ISBN 978-1-62873-647-2 (alk. paper)
1. Low-carbohydrate diet. 2. Natural foods. 3. Reducing diets--Recipes. 4. Weight loss. I. Title.
  RM237.73.P3818 2014
  613.2'833--dc23
                              2013044292

Printed in China

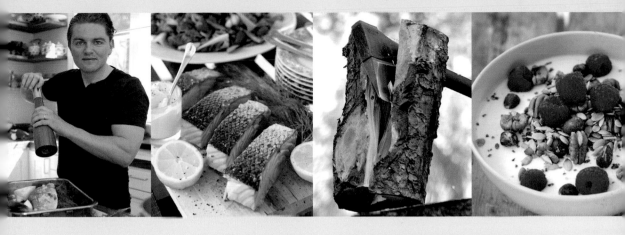

CONTENTS

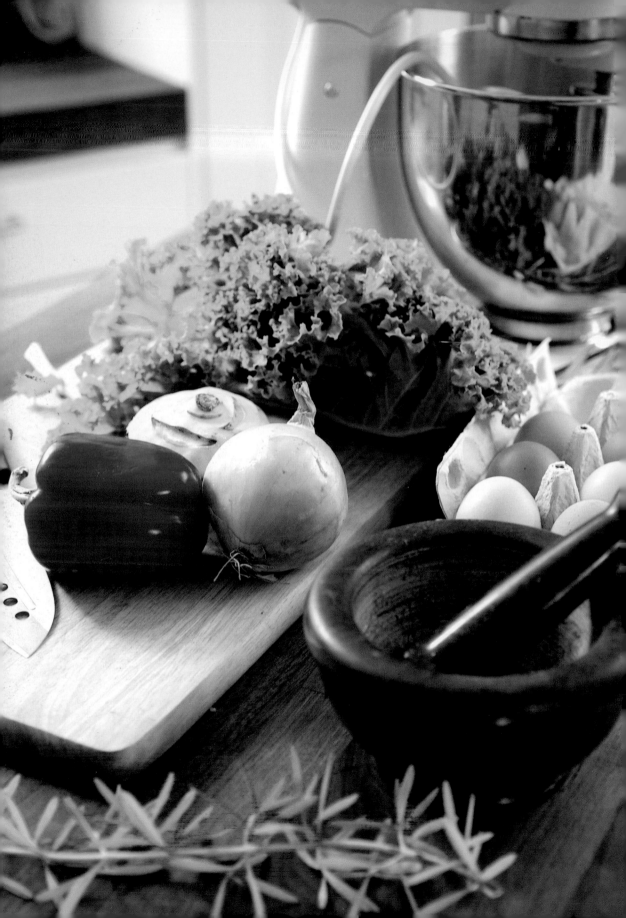

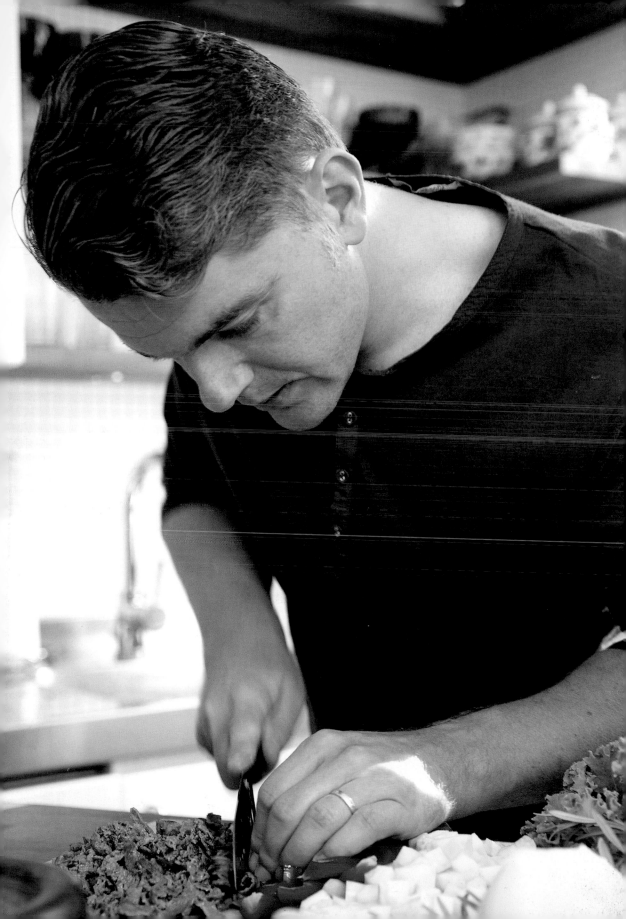

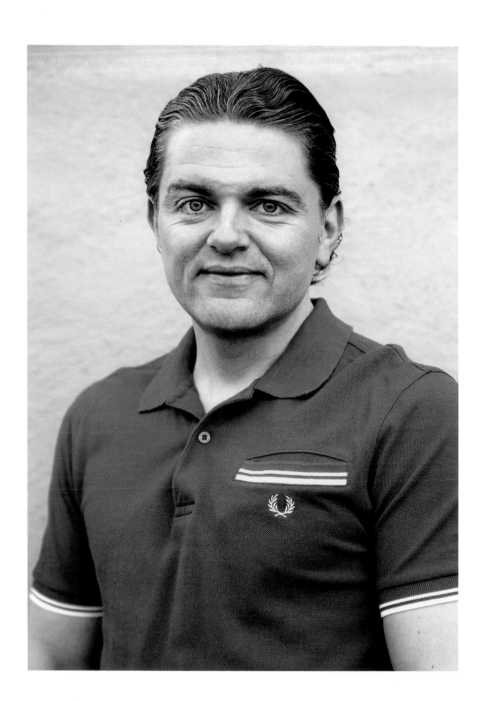

Introduction

"LCHQ is my interpretation of what constitutes the best food and what is the appropriate number of carbohydrates and kinds of fat you should eat."

When I more or less introduced the people of Sweden to the Glycemic Index in the late 1990s, one might say that the population was struck with carbohydrate fever. Or with fat phobia. This resulted in fat-free yogurts with more sugar than soda and other absurd products. Today we know better. Research and studies have advanced our knowledge. It's become evident that we should care not only about the Glycemic Index—fast- or slow-acting carbohydrates—but also about the number of carbohydrates in our food. The carbs we consume should, of course, be slow-acting, but most people would also benefit from reducing their intake of carbohydrates overall. That being said, it's just as unwise to eliminate all carbohydrates as it is to drastically reduce your intake of fat. The body is at its healthiest with a little bit of each, and this is exactly what the Low Carb High Quality (LCHQ) diet offers.

In the modern diet, there is one thing that predominates when it comes to causing disease and obesity: white sugar. The average American consumes way too much sugar, resulting in a surplus of energy and a nutrient deficiency. LCHQ helps eliminate sugar and prioritize nutritious food to strengthen rather than harm the body.

LCHQ is my interpretation of what constitutes the best food and what is the appropriate number of carbohydrates and kinds of fat you should eat. And, naturally, LCHQ is a lifestyle that promotes physical activity.

What Is LCHQ?

LCHQ is the abbreviation of Low Carb High Quality. It indicates a low-carb diet of high quality. High quality refers to both the quality of the food you eat, your experience of the food you eat, and how this affects your quality of life. Of course, food should provide you with energy, rather than drain energy from you. It should include enough nutrients to feed your muscles, brain, and immune system, as well as anything else that's fighting for the nutrients in your blood and cells. I'll describe the significance of that later in the book, but in general LCHQ is about reducing the number of carbohydrates in our diet without excluding them entirely.

Fat is a natural part of our diet, but it's not meant to be consumed in extreme amounts and the quality of the fat we do take in is very important. Some nutritionists recommend that you eat large amounts of animal fat, as they claim it doesn't harm your heart. In my opinion, this is misleading; there are plenty of other disadvantages to eating too much animal fat. For example, recent studies suggest that consuming too much animal fat reduces life expectancy and that saturated fat may increase the risk of cardiovascular disease (66). LCHQ was created to provide dieters with the right amount of fats that will burn fat, build muscle, reduce inflammations, and keep us healthy.

The protein intake in LCHQ is higher than what most people are used to, but it provides great health benefits, such as reduced blood pressure, increased muscle mass, and a better feeling of fullness or satisfaction after a meal.

This is not a diet that restricts caloric intake. It's a lifestyle that makes your body feel healthier and look better—without the anxiety that other diets often generate. LCHQ also includes exercise, because by simply moving your body and exercising your heart and other muscles, you can start feeling great. LCHQ is designed to be a lifestyle for the rest of your life.

CARBOHY-
DRATES

EXERCISE

PROTEIN   FAT

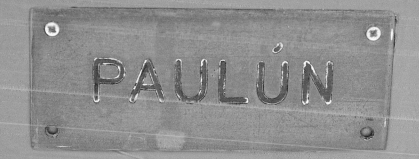

"Food should be enjoyed but not at the expense of your health."

What's behind LCHQ?

I have worked with dietetics for almost twenty years and I have a master's degree in nutrition. In plain English, this means that I'm a nutrition physiologist, and over the years I have met with and helped thousands of people. At Paulún's Nutrition Center, my staff and I have seen many people who feel fantastic as a result of following the LCHQ diet. Their blood lipids have improved, as well as their sensitivity to insulin. In general, they're able to sleep better and their mood is lighter now that they are making the choices that LCHQ promotes. Additionally, they tend to lose weight inadvertently, and the best part is that their body composition improves as a result of increased muscle mass. They are also left with the energy to exercise and they feel completely satisfied after each meal, which is incredibly important in order to maximize quality of life. No individual benefits from reducing his or her food intake over a long period of time, regardless of whether that means reducing portion size or simply omitting certain nutrients or foods that he or she actually enjoys.

I have firsthand experience of the benefits of LCHQ, and my own findings are supported by scholarly research that has been conducted on the topic. I have chosen a number of studies and will present them either in parenthesis at the end of my sentence or will reference them throughout the book. Please note that this is far from all the research that has been conducted on the subject; it is, however, a representative sampling.

My experience with LCHQ

I was born in 1970 and have been interested in various diets since the late 1980s. Since that time, I've tried pretty much every existing diet, including veganism, lacto veganism, the Stone Age diet, the junk food diet, fitness food, LCHF, low-fat diets, and everything in between. My goal has never been weight loss but simply to feel healthy and have enough energy for work, exercise, and leisure. Of course, I also have aesthetic and health reasons for keeping my body fat low. This is why my food needs to both maintain my quality of life and keep me in shape.

One can argue that LCHQ is a compilation of all of my favorite aspects of other diets. This is knowledge I have acquired over my years dieting and from the studies that I have read, and I am convinced that this is the optimal diet for us as humans.

By eating this way, I receive enough energy to exercise and plenty of nutrients for my cells. At the same time, I don't deprive myself of anything, nor do I suffer from either a surplus or a deficiency of any nutrients. This enables me to keep to the LCHQ diet as long as I want without any negative repercussions—something that is a risk with other diets. In fact, much of the LCHQ diet resembles the Stone Age diet, with a low caloric intake and an adequate intake of the right quality of fat.

Many of my colleagues in the nutrition industry stick to a diet that resembles LCHQ, and most people who exercise for aesthetic reasons do so as well. The former group follows this diet because LCHQ food is nutritious, whereas the latter do so because it's appropriate for building muscle and burning fat.

One of the biggest reasons why I like LCHQ is because of its versatility and vast array of ingredients. It's said that food should be enjoyed but not at the expense of your health. With this diet, I argue that you get both. This is why I believe you will like the LCHQ diet and will feel as great as I do if you follow it.

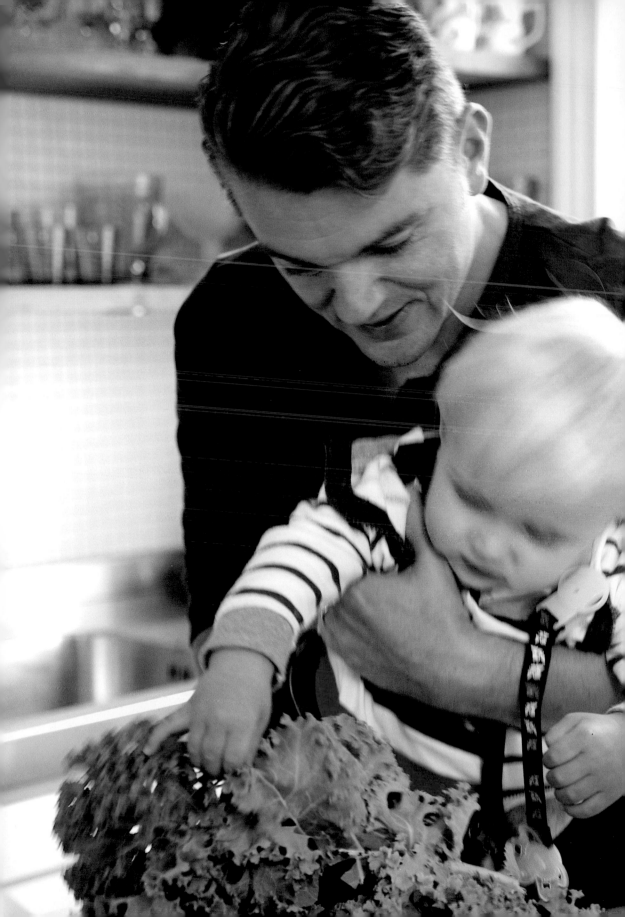

Carbohydrates: Quantity and Type

LCHQ is a diet with a considerably reduced average intake of carbohydrates—but it's not a minimal one. It's normal for LCHQ dieters to have about 20 E% (energy percent) carbohydrates (naturally these should be carbs with a low glycemic index). This means that about one-fifth of the energy comes from carbohydrates, and the rest from fat, protein, and possibly alcohol. The reduced number of slow-acting carbohydrates ensures a perfect blood sugar level between meals. And you'll be able to tell the difference. You will feel more alert than before because your brain will have constant access to blood sugar, and you won't become drowsy from the food. When you find yourself in a "lunch coma" after a calzone pizza, it's because your blood sugar rose too high in too short a period of time. This causes a too-rapid increase of the serotonin level in your brain, which in turn causes you to become drowsy. However, this doesn't happen with LCHQ. You might say that LCHQ food gives energy instead of draining it from you. Which is just how it should be.

Typical sources of carbohydrates for LCHQ dieters are nuts, seeds, vegetables, mushrooms, fruit, berries, root vegetables, and small amounts of rice, oats, quinoa, and corn. For those who benefit from a slightly higher intake of carbs, LCHQ allows for 30 E% from carbs, and then the remaining percent is divided up equally between fat and protein—i.e. 35 E% each. Everyone is different and some people need more in order to feel good, especially if they exercise a lot. During the weeks when I travel to health lectures, I exercise on a daily basis, which then means I need more carbohydrates. When it comes to my energy to work out, the difference is like night and day. Some days during these trips, I will load up on up to 30 E% of carbohydrates, resulting in a completely different level of stamina. It's still considerably lower than the 40 E% from carbs the average person consumes per day. Of course, how much food is consumed is also crucial for determining the total nutritional intake. But since you generally eat more when you exercise, this results in consuming more grams of everything.

LCHQ CARBOHYDRATES

- Vegetables
- Root vegetables (especially those with a low carb content)
- Nuts and seeds
- Fruit and berries, in moderation
- Small amounts of bulgur, quinoa, and brown rice

What happens when you don't eat enough carbohydrates?

As a result of today's general fear of carbohydrates, many people believe "the fewer the better." However, this is completely misguided. It's very risky to eliminate carbohydrates entirely from your body, since carbs are your body's primary fuel. If your blood contains glucose, this is primarily what the brain will use. During periods of starvation—or when you drastically reduce your intake of carbohydrates—the ketone production in your liver increases. Ketones are formed by fat and can be used by the brain when the glucose levels are insufficient, resulting in a state of ketosis. However, ketone is a backup fuel and the body reacts negatively when it's in a state of ketosisis for too long (18, 19, 21, 22, 23, 24). One thing that will result is that the body will want to reserve as much glucose as possible for the brain—and the only way to do so is to decrease sensitivity to insulin. The effect is that the insulin will not work as well in the muscles, liver, and kidneys (in other words, the insulin's effect as a "door opener" to the cells deteriorates), which can have extremely adverse consequences. At its worst, this can lead to type 2 diabetes, a disease that many people try to avoid by decreasing their intake of carbohydrates. Sure, an individual with type 2 diabetes can quickly reduce his or her blood sugar to a minimum by not consuming any carbs at all. The downside is that the disease worsens if you simply mask the symptoms. If a diabetic is not prepared to live the rest of his or her life without carbohydrates, he or she risks dangerously high blood sugar levels if he or she eats a high-carb meal. The best thing for someone with diabetes is to considerably reduce their the intake of carbs, but not exclude carbs entirely. Many foods with a high carbohydrate content, such as fruits, berries, vegetables, root vegetables, nuts, whole grain products, etc., all have health benefits for other reasons.

This is why LCHQ includes 20 E% of high quality carbohydrates. This is enough to keep the blood sugar in check without developing a resistance to insulin.

What about the ketones?

The fewer carbs you eat, the more ketones the body produces. But this is not an on or off function; rather, the ketone level changes gradually. For example, after a good night's sleep, we all have an elevated ketone level—even those who eat plenty of carbs.

When you follow the LCHQ diet, you will be in a mild state of ketosis, which is beneficial for many reasons. A certain state of ketosis makes it easier for your body to burn fat and maintain your weight. However, an intense state of ketosis (in other words, that which you achieve when you starve yourself or omit carbs entirely) is problematic in many ways. Ketones contain low levels of pH, so your body becomes more acidic (18, 19), which can increase your risk for osteoporosis (21, 22, 23) and inflammations (24).

LCHQ can make you happier

Excluding all carbohydrates from your diet can have a negative effect on your mood and quality of life. When your blood receives glucose, the brain creates serotonin, which makes you happy and satisfied! Research has shown that people who lose weight with a diet that prohibits carbs consider themselves less happy than people who have lost an equal amount of weight and were allowed to eat carbohydrates (20). In this respect, LCHQ is optimal. You consume enough carbs to keep up serotonin production, and you eat regularly, which maintains serotonin levels throughout the day. Another important factor is that LCHQ includes the right types of fat to make you feel better mentally and emotionally. It also contains high levels of omega-3 fats and research has shown that these increase the brain's ability to regulate serotonin. In this way, omega-3 decreases the risk of depression and may, in fact, help mitigate it.

The right quantity of carbs provides energy and motivation to exercise

A certain intake of carbs is also important to the LCHQ lifestyle, because I promote exercise. You never feel as good as when you devote yourself to physical activity.

The more ketones you have, the less you'll want to exercise. The LCHQ diet balances ketones and glucose perfectly, giving you enough energy for both your muscles and your brain. It's not surprising that the body indicates fatigue when it's in a state of ketosis, since ketones appear during starvation—signaling to the body that it needs to save as much energy as possible. The 20 E% of carbs in LCHQ are enough to make the body feel as though it has enough energy to exercise and increase the fat-burning process. Because LCHQ contains a high intake of protein, it's an optimal diet for building muscle. This is important for people of all ages, but especially for older generations, who often suffer from reduced muscle mass and strength, or sarcopenia. It's a serious condition, which increases the risk of falling, disease, and premature death. Therefore, eating LCHQ foods paired with reasonable exercise is an effective strategy for both the young and the elderly who want to improve their physique for a long, healthy life. As previously mentioned, I have personally tried almost every type of diet, and I know if

I consume fewer carbs than are suggested by LCHQ, my ketone levels will rise too high. This means that my desire to exercise will decrease and I won't achieve the active lifestyle that leads to the quality of life I want.

LCHQ's low glycemic index keeps you young

All natural foods that contain carbohydrates slowly elevate your blood sugar. Your body was designed to handle this process. If you instead eat too many fast-acting carbohydrates, you will feel bad and might get sick. Such foods can harm your body and may cause you to age more quickly and suffer from cardiovascular disease. It's also evident that such food has the ability to be stored in your body as fat. By avoiding such a diet, you can easily decrease your body fat. I'm sure you already know that fast-acting carbohydrates exist in things like white sugar, instant mashed potatoes, sugary cereals, soda, and white flour products.

Naturally, LCHQ only includes carbs with a low glycemic index. You'll probably notice it in the form of a quicker fat-burning process and a stronger mental performance. You won't notice that you are simultaneously reducing your risk of a heart attack. Type 2 diabetes and many tumor diseases also correlate with a high glycemic index, so hopefully your retirement won't include any of these things.

Something that you will probably notice decades after having maintained a low GI diet is that you're able to age with dignity. Because you avoided the glycation that accompanies high blood sugar (sugar molecules bind with protein or fat, which decreases their functionality in the body), you won't suffer from the stiffness or high blood pressure that usually comes with old age. You'll probably also look younger than your friends who have kept a high GI diet, since age-related skin deterioration actually stems from glycated collagen, and is therefore caused by a high glycemic index. Even reduced brain functionality can be related to glycation, because dementia includes elevated levels of glycated proteins in the brain.

Free from refined sugar

It probably hasn't been lost on anyone that Americans consume high volumes of added and refined sugar. Approximately one out of every five calories consumed in this country comes from added sugar. All this sugariness makes one's blood sugar skyrocket, harming the body's proteins. In an attempt to reduce the blood sugar level, the body releases insulin, which causes such side effects as the storing of fat, increased blood fat, and insulin resistance.

We also know that sugar and sweeteners tend to increase our appetite and make us crave even more sweetness. Think about your own life: Do you ever have periods where you have an elevated desire for sweet foods? If you eat candy for a couple of days straight, it begins to take incredible willpower to go without sugar. But once you've been without sugar for a couple of days, this desire for sweetness will lessen and lessen until it is virtually gone.

LCHQ is, of course, free from all refined sugar. There's simply no room for candy or other sweets if a maximum of 20 E% is supposed to come from carbohydrates. However, what can fit are fresh or frozen fruits and berries. These taste sweet but they contain natural sugar, as well as thousands of healthy nutrients, such as fibers, antioxidants, vitamins, and minerals. Therefore, in its natural form, sugar is actually nutritious. Additionally, fruits and berries contain extremely few calories. They consist of about 80 to 90 percent water, making them very filling in relation to their low calorie levels.

Dried fruit is also healthy, but it contains a few too many carbs and concentrated energy to be included in LCHQ. Dried berries are better, but watch out for the sweetened ones!

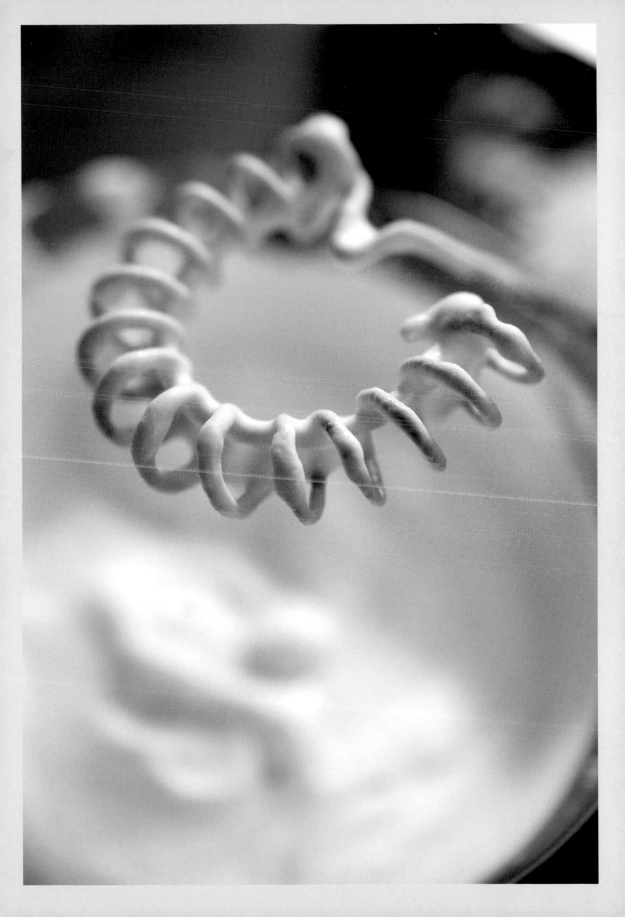

LCHQ is anti-inflammatory

Your body is host to a constant battle between substances that cause inflammations and those that prevent inflammations. Inflammations are necessary; they constitute an important part of your immune system and ensure that tissue can heal. If you exercise a lot, an inflammatory response is needed in order to recover from the workout and achieve the desired results. However, if an inflammation becomes too severe, you'll get sick, and it may increase your risk of cancer, cardiovascular disease, type 2 diabetes, and autoimmune disease.

Pain is almost always due to inflammation, and if you suffer from chronic pain, chances are that the pain will mitigate if you reduce the chance of inflammations.

Interestingly, you can affect inflammations through your diet. A high intake of carbohydrates, especially fast-acting ones, increases the inflammations in your body. LCHQ promotes a balance of nutrients and ingredients that keep inflammation in check without eliminating them entirely. Many people suffer from too many inflammations, so you may notice a positive effect when beginning the LCHQ diet. A reduced number of headaches is a good example, as well as decreased flare-ups of eczema and joint pain. What also makes the LCHQ diet effective against inflammation is that it contains fruit, berries, and vegetables, all of which contain high quantities of naturally anti-inflammatory nutrients (45). Additionally, the LCHQ diet includes fish, nuts, red wine, olive oil, and regular exercise, and these are also known to be anti-inflammatory. It's also beneficial that LCHQ food is cooked at a low temperature, and it lessens the consumption of meat from cattle and livestock (read more on page 37).

A low glycemic index and the right number of carbs are therefore very important here.

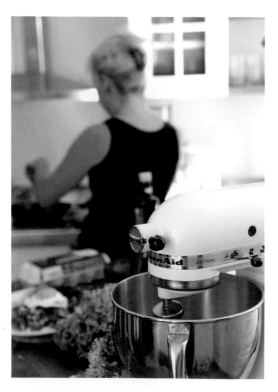
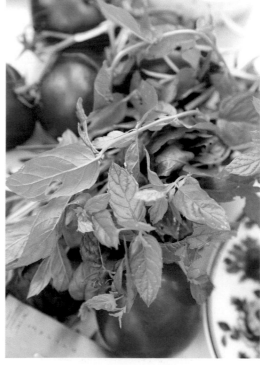

LCHQ for Weight Loss

LCHQ is in itself not a diet for achieving weight loss; instead, it's a lifestyle. With LCHQ, you can eat a wide array of food and can essentially have as much of it as you like—as long as the food is of the right quality. However, LCHQ is perfect for losing weight, and if weight loss is the goal rather than a healthy lifestyle, it becomes known as the "iso diet." It is well proven and provides some amazing results without being too strenuous. Most people on the iso diet lose 1.8–3.3 lbs (0.8–1.5 kg) per week while consuming all necessary nutrients without any deficiencies; this enables them to achieve their target weight. The iso diet provides 33 E% of fat, protein, and carbohydrates respectively, which results in a daily intake of 1600 calories. Because the iso diet relies on pre-made menus, it's truly easy to follow and most dieters think they get more than enough to eat. Quite simply, they get full and stay full. This is because the iso diet relies on the most filling foods per calorie. It also calls for food with a low glycemic index, which has a proven effective on one's sense of satiety. Protein intake is high, which is not only filling, but also increases fat burning and energy expenditure. In the spirit of LCHQ, the fat that is consumed is of the highest quality with a focus on unsaturated fat and short/medium saturated fats. A low intake of long-chain saturated fats helps keep body fat low.

20 or 33 E% carbohydrates?

A frequent question that iso dieters ask is why they should have a higher energy intake from carbohydrates compared to LCHQ. The iso diet demands 33 E% carbohydrates, whereas LCHQ only requires 20 E%. The answer is that when you count the total number of calories, it's pretty much the same for each diet. The iso diet has a standard caloric intake of 1600 calories per day, and with 33 E% from carbs, this means that approximately 528 calories

come from carbs. Because each gram of carbohydrates constitutes 4 calories, this means that the iso diet allows you 130 grams of carbohydrates. With LCHQ, you're allowed to eat without restrictions, and you don't follow a particular diet, since it's not technically a weight loss diet (this is what the iso diet is for). But LCHQ fills you up and will likely generate some weight loss. With LCHQ, you may actually eat around 2,500 calories a day, and if 20 percent of them come from carbs, this means about 500 calories from carbs a day. This corresponds to 125 grams of carbs—almost identical to the iso diet. This means that both diets provide you with enough energy for the brain, muscles, immune system, and other parts of your body that rely on carbs for fuel. However, the iso diet restricts the number of calories to provide effective weight loss.

" Most people on the iso diet lose 1.8–3.3 lbs (0.8–1.5 kg) per week."

Protein: Meat, Fish, or Poultry?

When it comes to today's popular diets, there are any number of letter combinations. But it's imperative that you understand the difference between them. LCHP denotes Low Carb High Protein and promotes a high intake of protein from which the majority of the diet's energy stems. This method has been used for decades by bodybuilders and fitness lovers who really want to minimize their body fat. LCHP works really well for this purpose; however, I don't think it's a good diet for the long term. Sure, protein is better than most substances at providing a high feeling of fullness per calorie (32) and it increases the number of fat-burning hormones. It also costs a lot of energy to break down protein, which increases energy expenditure. Therefore, protein is almost magical for quickly reducing body fat. It also builds and/or saves muscle tissue, which is incredibly effective for preventing disease and shaping an attractive physique.

But in the long run, such a high intake of protein is not desirable. First of all, it's not particularly enjoyable to eat only cod and vegetables or grilled chicken with a glass of water. Secondly, you risk eating too few fatty acids. LCHQ gives you 30 to 40 E% of protein, which is more than enough for getting all the health benefits, but it also allows for 40 to 50 E% worth of fat. This means you'll consume all the important fatty acids and will continue burning fat. As you might deduce, the body burns the nutrients it is fed; so if you eat fat, you'll also burn fat.

What happens when you eat 30–40 E% percent worth of protein?

First of all, 30–40 E% is not an extreme amount, but it is considerably higher than what the average American consumes. Today's normal protein intake is around 15 E%.

Secondly, it is possible to cook really delicious food using chicken, fish, seafood, eggs, and lean meat. Even dairy products can work well as long as the fat content is reasonable and the protein level is high. Cottage cheese, quark, yogurt, and lean cheeses are all great sources of protein.

The first thing you will notice about the LCHQ diet is that you will achieve a greater sense of satiety after meals than usual. It's not as aggressive a fullness as the feeling you get after eating a lot of fat. Instead, it's a pleasantly satisfied feeling that lasts for a long time. The protein ensures that your stomach is emptied slower, allowing for a more gradual increase in blood sugar.

Can too much protein have adverse effects?

Can a high intake of protein be potentially harmful? If you're in general good health, the answer is no. If you have bad kidneys, their function might suffer more from an increased intake of protein, but for a healthy individual there is virtually no risk. The kidneys have a large capacity that can in theory handle all the calories consumed through protein.

An old myth is that a high protein intake acidifies the body and increases the level of calcium in the urine. It was believed that the skeleton simply releases calcium to counteract the acidification believed to be caused by the protein. However, when you examine the bone density of people who consume a lot of protein, the complete opposite appears to be true! Increased protein intake seems to increase the calcium uptake in the small intestine, which admittedly increases the calcium level in the urine but also in the skeletal structure. Thus, a high protein intake prevents osteoporosis (31).

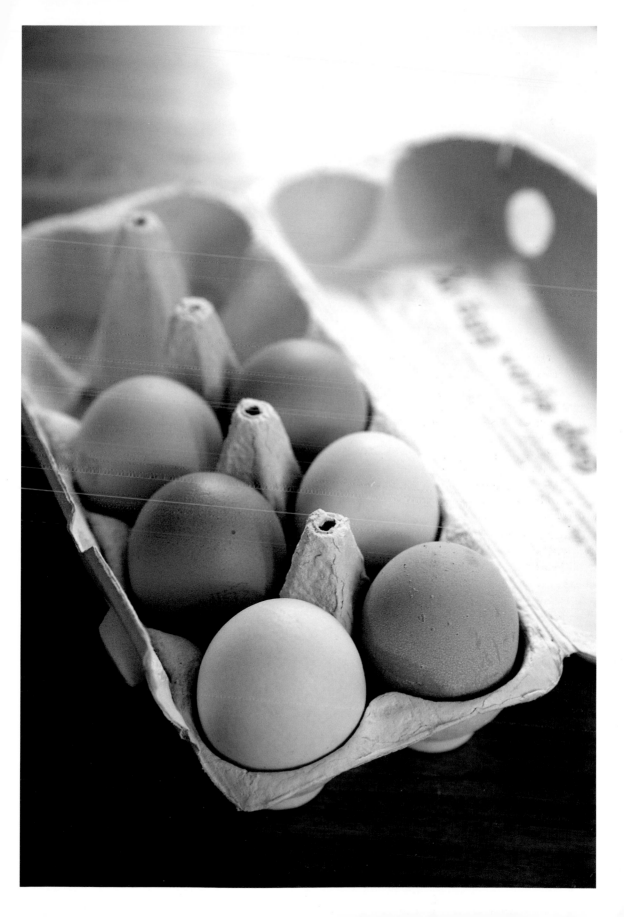

Maximize Antioxidants

LCHQ food is naturally rich in antioxidants— ingredients that can easily be summed up as your elixir of life. If you didn't have antioxidants in your body, you would not be alive for very long. In proof of this, there are some genetic diseases that cause an inability to produce certain antioxidants, thereby reducing life expectancy significantly.

Your body receives antioxidants both of its own production and from the food that you eat—at least, it will if you eat the proper food. In fact, such "proper" food is often considered healthy precisely because of its high level of antioxidants. Berries, fruits, vegetables, nuts, legumes, seeds, cold pressed oils, root vegetables, mushrooms, game, fish, seafood, spices, herbs, tea, coffee, chocolate, and red wine are all extremely good sources of antioxidants.

Antioxidants protect your proteins from oxidizing, which ensures that the bad cholesterol LDL (which predominantly consists of protein) doesn't go rancid and get stuck in your blood vessels. In this way, you avoid heart attacks. This also protects your DNA, thereby reducing your risk for cancer and premature aging. Your immune system works more effectively if your body contains antioxidants, and as a special bonus, they're anti-inflammatory. Many antioxidants are also described as having the ability to widen your blood vessels, thereby keeping your blood pressure low.

Optimal absorbance

Antioxidants exist in large quantities and have varying characteristics. This is why it's important to include a large number of various vegetables in your cooking, which fortunately happens to be one of the main aspects of the LCHQ diet.

Some antioxidants are sensitive to heat, but most of them handle it pretty well. Boiling the vegetables or making a stir fry is generally fine. Sometimes the uptake of antioxidants is improved by the cooking process. Changing the structure of the antioxidants makes them easier to digest, which in turn makes it easier for your body to absorb the nutrients. Since many antioxidants are fat-soluble and food usually contains fat, the antioxidants follow the fat into the body.

You shouldn't cook food so long that it changes color due to the heat. This only results in a loss of antioxidants; the browned or "ruined" food surface actually indicates lost nutrition.

Which vegetables are the most sensitive?

Depending on how you measure the level of antioxidants and how you cook the food, the results tend to vary. I have specifically focused on one study that examined several vegetables that were boiled, cooked in the microwave, cooked in a pressure-cooker, fried, griddled, and baked in the oven. The artichokes were tough, and did not lose a significant number of antioxidants regardless of how they were cooked. The most sensitive vegetables were the boiled and microwaved cauliflowers, boiled peas, and boiled and fried zucchini. Beets, green beans, and garlic retained most of their antioxidants regardless of how they were cooked. Bell peppers lost some antioxidants in all the different methods of cooking, whereas celery actually increased its antioxidant content unless it was boiled, upon which it lost about 14 percent of its antioxidants. Even carrots benefited from being cooked, and they certainly improve a Bolognese sauce.

Are you wondering which cooking method was best for maintaining the level of antioxidants? Griddling, microwaving, and baking in the oven. These allowed the vegetables to maintain their initial levels of antioxidants the best, whereas pressure-cooking and boiling caused the highest loss of antioxidants. This may seem surprising, but it's predominantly due to the fact that the boiling water pretty much drains the vegetables (30).

Tricks for increasing the antioxidant content

There are several ways to increase the level of antioxidants in the body and also to consume the right types of antioxidants. The easiest and most obvious trick is to include high-antioxidant foods in every meal, and be sure to vary the colors of the foods. Different colors indicate different types of antioxidants, and the more types you consume the better you will feel.

Research has found that you're less likely to have damaged DNA if you consume ten serv ings of 100 grams of different vegetables per day than if you have a portion of, for example, one kilogram of broccoli. New studies also show that you should avoid pouring milk into your tea because this reduces access to healthy flavonoids (27). Interestingly, skim milk was the worst offender, so if you want milk in your tea, you should use milk with a high fat content. However, even those had a negative effect. It is unclear whether or not this also holds true for coffee, but I would assume so.

Because many antioxidants are fat-soluble, it's good to consume a certain amount of fat along with the antioxidants. A sliced tomato topped with olive oil can enable you to absorb twice as many antioxidants as when you eat the tomato by itself.

Frozen antioxidants are super effective

Sometimes it's difficult to find superfoods in the produce aisle. Sure, there are often blueberries, raspberries, and blackberries in the fruit section, but these are often over-priced and nearing their expiration date.

The same is true for super-healthy vegetables like broccoli or asparagus. The solution is the freezer aisle. Here, you'll find the superfoods listed above, as well as several specialized products, including small packets of frozen acai puree. Acai puree is made from the Brazilian superberry that contains incredible quantities of antioxidants. It's a great ingredient in smoothies or homemade ice cream.

The best thing about freezing is that the process is gentle toward antioxidants. Research has shown that most of the antioxidants will remain in the foods as long as they haven't expired (29). Since frozen produce is usually cheaper, I consider it a great bargain in terms of nutrition and cost.

"Different colors indicate different types of antioxidants, and the more types you consume the better you will feel."

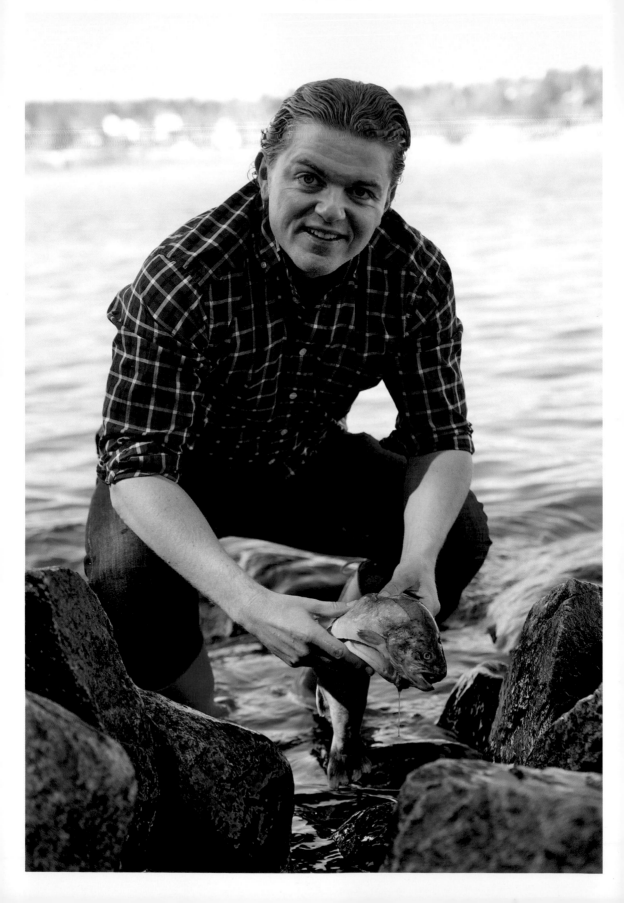

Fat: Saturated or Unsaturated?

Fat is arguably the most important nutrient to consume in order to feel good and function properly. Fat builds our bodies because it's included in our cell membranes. Fat also ensures that we can absorb the nutrients in fat-soluble vitamins and antioxidants. We also know that the body prefers to burn the nutrients that we feed it, so if you consume only low amounts of fat, your fat-burning process will suffer. A reasonable amount of fat will also make you feel full longer, keeping your faculties sharp and preventing weight gain. Basically, we have to consume the proper amounts and types of fat.

At the same time, you shouldn't eat too much fat. It will make you gain weight. There are twice as many calories in fat as in carbohydrates and protein. A fat intake that is too high will cause inflammations in your body, because it will stimulate the uptake of endotoxins in your intestines. Endotoxins are toxins that are produced by bacteria in the intestines and are fat-soluble, which causes the level of endotoxins in your blood to increase by as much as 50 percent. This generates inflammation and is harmful to your health. Balance is the key word here, which is exactly what LCHQ provides. 40 E% of fat is not much more than the average person consumes, so you may not have to make any significant change to your daily fat consumption. However, you should keep an eye on the quality of the fats consumed, because this is key in order for the fats to function properly.

LCHQ and the quality of the fat

Food contains saturated, monounsaturated, and polyunsaturated fat. Each has a special function and you shouldn't be afraid of any of them. However, research has shown that there is a certain fat composition that is optimal for humans. It basically focuses on monounsaturated fat, which protects you from cardiovascular disease and type 2 diabetes, as well as many forms of cancer. Good sources of monounsaturated fat are olive oil, avocado, nuts, and canola oil, to name a few. In fact, most sources of fat contain monounsaturated fat.

Polyunsaturated fat is also good for your cardiovascular health and can be derived from plant sources, such as seeds, grains, oats, and legumes, as well as from fish and seafood. Even some nuts have a relatively high content of polyunsaturated fat. It's also this fat, along with short and medium-long saturated fats, that the body is best able to process.

The short and medium-long saturated fats can be found in dairy products and coconut oil, and are included in the LCHQ diet. Research has actually shown that these are great for maintaining your weight and overall health, and they are also stable, which means that they don't suffer the risk of going rancid in your body.

LCHQ vs LCHF

A couple of years ago, the Swedish diet Low Carb High Fat (LCHF) started gaining national attention. In simple terms, LCHF is one of the most extreme diets that has ever existed. It basically restricts your intake of carbohydrates to 5–10 E% per day and replaces the lost carbs with large quantities of fat. Bacon, lard, cream, and butter were staples for this diet—and I consciously chose the past tense because LCHF has since become less strict and more varied in recent years. Today, some LCHF proponents recommend that you eat fruit, berries, and other fats in addition to the saturated fats, which I find to be a beneficial and healthy development. Many recent LCHF cookbooks contain some great recipes. I'm not critical of today's more commercial interpretation of LCHF, which is sometimes referred to as "liberal LCHF."

I am, however, very critical of the original form of LCHF. Strict LCHF (I'll call it "classic LCHF") is based on saturated animal fat, which has proven to be very unhealthy in myriad ways. An important thing to note here is that not all types of saturated fat were created equal. They exist in different forms, and research has shown that the short and medium saturated fats are good for your weight and your overall health. Many studies also show that they serve to improve your ability to burn fat and expend energy while also maintaining your weight (33–42). Short and medium saturated fats constitute about 60 to 70 percent of the fat in coconut and palm oil, 25 percent of the fat in dairy, and it is commonly found in breast milk. It's the long-chain saturated fats found in lard and fatty meat products that cause such health issues as type 2 diabetes and cardiovascular disease (66).

When I refer to LCHF in this book, I mean the extreme form that recommends a minimal intake of carbs and an extreme consumption of long-chain saturated fat. I am fully aware that there are healthier versions of LCHF ("liberal LCHF"), and I have nothing against them, although I do believe that LCHQ is the best option for most people.

Here is the scientific understanding of LCHQ and classic LCHF:

The quality of fat in LCHQ is beneficial for reducing oxidative stress. After each meal, the free radicals in your body increase and LCHQ, with its high content of monounsaturated fat, trumps that of LCHF. One study showed that people who consumed monounsaturated fat for twelve weeks had less oxidized fat in their bodies than those who consumed long-chain saturated fat (1).

You will probably live longer if you eat LCHQ rather than classic LCHF. A very large study (of approximately 130,000 people) showed that a low-carb diet that was based on animal products resulted in a shorter life expectancy than a low-carb diet combined with vegetable foodstuffs. Following the animal product-based diet results in a much higher consumption of long-chain saturated fats, while the vegetable-based diet results in the consumption of more unsaturated fats. The overall mortality rate increased, regardless of whether you examined cancer, cardiovascular disease, strokes, or other diseases (2). LCHQ encourages the consumption of many more vegetables, which provide much more than just the healthy fats. Vegetables also contain more antioxidants, phytonutrients, and fibers.

Your heart also benefits more from LCHQ than from LCHF. If you study the research, it's evident that reducing the consumption of long-chain saturated fat in favor of unsaturated fat reduced the risk of cardiovascular disease (3). You can experience dramatic effects if you increase your healthy fat consumption by an ounce (28.35 g) of nuts and exclude the equivalent amount of calories of saturated fats (which is a typical effect of LCHQ). This decreases the risk for cardiovascular disease by 45 percent (4)! Research also shows that too high an intake of fat (regardless of quality) reduces the amount of available energy for the heart muscle, resulting in a very dangerous situation for people suffering from heart failure (46).

Ⓠ Pertaining to the risk of cancer, research shows that saturated fat increases the risk of breast cancer (5, 6), ovarian cancer (7), and lymphoma (8). Personally, I think that studies that point to a certain type of nutrient as the cause of disease sometimes suggest that the root of the problem is actually a low intake of other nutrients. A high intake of saturated fat is almost always an automatic indicator of a low intake of omega-3 and omega-9 fats, which seem to reduce the risk of cancer.

Therefore, I don't think that a reasonable consumption of long-chain saturated fat is dangerous in this regard, but it does push out other necessary fats. And this is exactly what happens with LCHF, since the high intake of long-chain saturated fat leads to a very one-sided and unhealthy diet.

Ⓠ You will lose weight much faster and more effectively if you skip long-chain saturated fats in favor of the unsaturated fat advocated in LCHQ. One study showed that LCHQ, with more unsaturated fat from fish, seafood, and chicken, generated 1.1 lbs (.5 kg) more weight lost during a four-week period, compared to an LCHF diet consisting of fat from livestock that had been fattened with concentrates (9). Generally speaking, long-chain saturated fat is the most fattening thing that exists, except for synthetic trans fats.

Ⓠ Your brain is healthier when you consume reasonable amounts of fat and carbohydrates. Research shows that a diet with 75 E% fat causes a diminished attention span and mood, and makes your thought process slower compared to a diet of 23 E% fat (46). Another study shows that weight loss through LCHF results in

aggression and hostility toward one's environment (47). Based on my personal experience, I can testify to how a lack of carbs affects one's mood, and I have run into several angry LCHF proponents over the years. This same research shows that LCHF users become more and more depressed while adhering to the diet, which is problematic because life is too short to be unhappy.

Ⓠ LCHF with low levels of carbs and a lot of animal fat increases the risk for type 2 diabetes, whereas LCHQ, with low levels of carbs and much higher levels of vegetable fat, prevents it (47).

"An important thing to note here is that not all types of saturated fat were created equal."

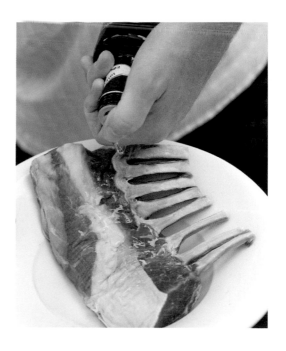

"If the color of your food has changed due to heat, you've created unhealthy types of fat."

Free from trans fats

Trans fats have a proven harmful effect on your heart and blood vessels. It also affects growth in children, and lowers infant birth weight if consumed while pregnant. It also increases the risk for cancer and makes inflammations more aggressive; this all adds up to mean that trans fats are one of few components in food that you should avoid at all costs. Luckily, most countries have placed a restriction on the level of trans fats that food is allowed to contain, and some states and cities in the United States have actively banned trans fats. However, imported products from other countries may not adhere to these standards. Trans fats can also arise from cooking your food.

Because trans fats are created from fat being heated up or industrially cured, they're pretty simple to avoid. One method is to simply cook food at reasonable temperatures. Avoid deep frying anything, and avoid creating a fried surface on your food. If the color of your food has changed due to heat, you've created unhealthy types of fat and destroyed the carbohydrates and proteins, which will negatively affect your health. Generally speaking, frying should occur at low temperatures and with fats that can withstand heat, such as olive oil, avocado oil, or better yet, coconut oil.

The food industry has enjoyed putting trans fats in all types of products, because trans fats are inexpensive to produce and long-lasting. Trans fats give cheaply-made food a better taste and texture. Unfortunately, it's not always easy to detect "trans fat" on the nutritional label, since it doesn't always go by that name. It's often indicated by the phrase "partially hydrogenated oils," which could, for example, be canola oil that has been exposed to high temperatures, hydrogen gas, and a catalyst such as nickel. This process saturates the fatty acids, and eventually, the oil will consist solely of saturated fat and will be basically useless because it has been so completely hardened. Therefore, the hardening process is halted after a while, resulting in a fat that is semi-liquid, durable, and contains lethal trans fats.

Thankfully, many companies have eliminated trans fats from their products. However, they still often show up in finished goods, candy, pastries, snacks, frying oils, etc. This is why you should avoid products that include "partially hydrogenated oil," "hydrogenated fat," "partially hydrogenated fat," or "hardened oil." Sometimes it says "hardened" instead of hydrogenated, but it's the same thing. When you eat LCHQ, your food should generally be of a high quality, which automatically excludes trans fats.

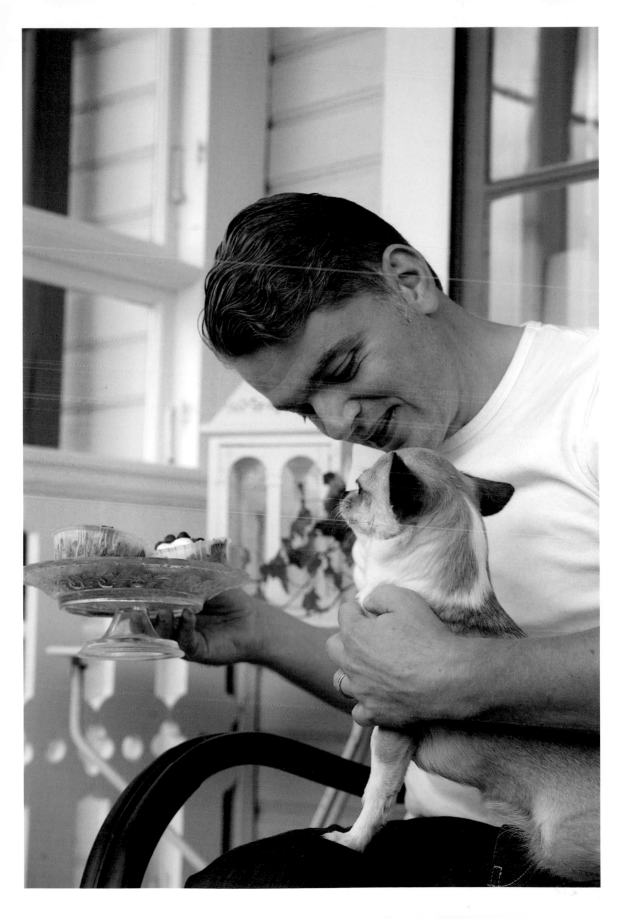

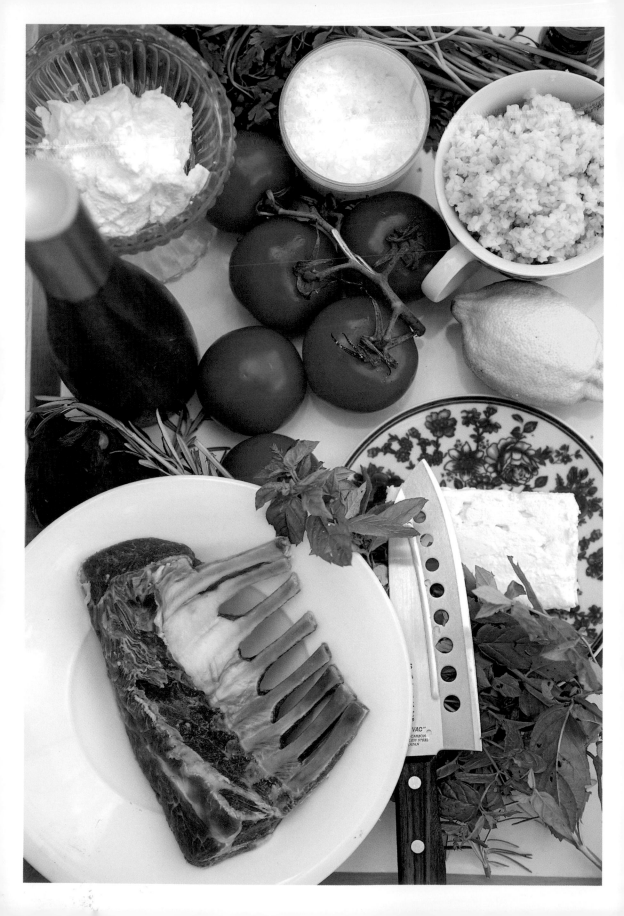

LCHQ Is Real Food

By real food, I mean food that relies on fresh, raw ingredients, not semi-finished products or chemicals. Many people eat fake food without thinking about it: instant sauces, frozen hamburgers, cheese doodles, corn flakes, and vitamin waters. These are examples of foods that have been created with various chemicals and components that make the concoction taste like food, look like food, and smell like food—but in my opinion, it isn't food. These are made of additives, extracts, and refined products. For example, corn flakes are made from cornmeal that has been roasted so hard that you have to add vitamins and minerals to them in order for them to contain anything but quick carbs. Instant sauces are made from starch, fat, scents, and other additives that make it taste like gravy, but it isn't actually gravy at all. In my opinion, it's much better to make homemade, creamy sauce than buy a powder—even if the calorie content of your version is higher. Vitamin drinks are often just vitamin-infused sugar water. Frozen hamburgers and sausage often contain way too much fat, because it's a cheap component compared to the protein. LCHQ relies on real food, real ingredients, and real nutrients.

Real food takes some planning

In order to cook real food, you'll need to have access to the right ingredients. This means the vegetable cubby in the refrigerator should be kept well-stocked. Of course, it's fine to purchase pre-washed bags of lettuce that can be placed on a plate and drizzled with some olive oil. This type of "ready-made" food is composed of real ingredients and is good for you. You don't even have to have fresh produce all the time. Frozen produce is great—it's not like the frozen meat products that are stuffed with a bunch of additives. Be sure to shop for bargains and keep your freezer stocked with fish, seafood, vegetables, chicken, and beef. Some canned foods are great too, as long as they hold somewhat organic ingredients, such as tuna or crushed tomatoes. These are largely the same as their fresh counterparts.

With a little planning, you'll soon discover that it's easy to keep pantry, fridge, and freezer well stocked with high-quality, real food.

Minimal use of additives

I'm not particularly afraid of additives, since most of them have been extensively researched and deemed to be harmless. Some additives can even be healthy! Alginates are a good example; these are water-soluble fibers that stem from algae. Water-soluble fibers reduce the glycemic index of your food and provide your digestive system with probiotics (see page 31). Even the blood fats improve, so the right additives can really be beneficial. Despite this, LCHQ food contains very few additives because you cook most of the food from scratch. Or at least, you "build" your food from organic ingredients. This way you can also avoid most harmful additives.

Flavor enhancers, for example, can increase your appetite and contribute to weight gain. Color dyes and preservatives can negatively affect your ability to concentrate. Modified starch is a chemically altered form of starch that can be oxidized. Oxidized fat and protein have been demonstrated to be harmful, so oxidized starch is hardly a healthy thing to consume.

Even your sodium level is automatically regulated in the LCHQ diet, because LCHQ avoids ready-made food and additives, which often contain a lot of salt.

LCHQ is natural food, cooked on your terms, without additives.

LCHQ and probiotics

The only things it might be difficult to obtain through LCHQ food are probiotics—in other words, healthy bacteria. Despite the high quality of the ingredients, they generally contain small amounts of bacteria. Your intestines naturally contain many kinds if bacteria, all of which serve a different purpose in your body.

You can control your intestinal flora in part by taking supplements and in part by the food you eat. A healthy intestinal flora generates a stonger immune system, fewer allergic reactions and intolerances, a stronger stomach, fewer dental cavities, better breath, and a reduced risk for cardiovascular diseases and type 2 diabetes. It even reduces the risk for intestinal cancer. Recent studies have also found that a healthy intestinal flora can protect children against ADHD!

As you may have figured out, these microorganisms affect your whole body, so it's very important for your health to have an appropriate level of probiotics. Modern food contains very little bacteria. This includes both the healthy and unhealthy bacteria, and is a result of pasteurization, refrigeration, and preservation of food. Therefore, it's important that you actively seek out food with healthy bacteria cultures and take supplements. Throughout history, our ancestors have ingested healthy bacteria, and in order to optimize our own health, we need to follow in their footsteps.

How to come by probiotics
Due to the fact that the benefits of a healthy intestinal flora have been extensively researched and established by science, the food industry has begun adding healthy bacteria cultures to many products. Yogurt is one of the most natural options, since the bacteria actually participate in its making (you simply cannot make yogurt without bacteria). You should, of course, be sure to choose plain yogurt because otherwise it's not LCHQ.

More and more products are being enriched with probiotics, but unfortunately these are usually the refined and manufactured types of foods and are not always the best option. For example, they exist in many beverages that also contain sugar and various additives.

Personally, I have chosen to take a daily supplement of probiotics (Lactiplus) since 2005. Interestingly, I no longer get many colds, whereas before I took the supplement, I was afflicted with colds two to three times a year. I'm sure there are several other health benefits that I haven't noticed. For example, small inflammations of the intestines can be difficult to detect if there aren't other stomach issues to attract your notice, but in the long run these surely decrease. A supplement of probiotics is therefore something I recommend to everyone, including children and seniors. Other

*"Modern food contains very little bacteria.
This includes both the healthy and unhealthy bacteria,
and is a result of pasteurization, refrigeration,
and preservation of food."*

natural sources of probiotics are sauerkraut and cheese.

Probiotics are most effective when consumed year-round, but it is, of course, better to ingest them during short bursts than not at all. Some experts claim that you should take a supplement or eat a type of food with only one specific strain of bacteria, whereas others argue that a broader intake of diverse types of bacteria is better for health.

Personally, I agree with the latter method, since that's how man has historically consumed bacteria. I try to eat a wide array of different bacteria in order to receive a natural, diverse intake; this means I don't feel the need to switch out any supplements or foods that I eat.

High fiber content

LCHQ is naturally rich in fibers, which has an enormously positive effect on your health and quality of life. Among many things, fiber-rich food is very chewy, which has proven to be good for the brain. There appears to be a neurological connection between the teeth and the brain, so chewy food stimulates the brain. And chances are good that this will improve your

cognitive abilities. When the fibers land in your stomach, they provide a heightened sense of satiety. When the fibers reach the small intestine, they fill you up even more and improve your digestive function. The movement of your intestines is more effective when they have something to work with.

It is customary to distinguish between water-soluble and water-insoluble fibers, which have different characteristics. Water-soluble fibers exist predominantly in fruit, berries, legumes, seeds, vegetables, and certain grains and have really interesting qualities. They balance your blood sugar while simultaneously improving your blood (these effects occur in the small intestine). Water-insoluble fibers are the colon bacteria's favorite fuel, and they provide these healthy bacteria with the energy boost they need to grow.

Water-insoluble fibers are probiotic, meaning they are the fuel for your healthy bacteria. They allow for a strong intestinal flora with a well-functioning stomach and strong immune system.

The water-insoluble fibers are also good for the digestive system, but they do not offer the same health benefits for the blood sugar, intestinal flora, etc. LCHQ includes not only an adequate amount of fiber, but also a high amount of water-soluble fibers.

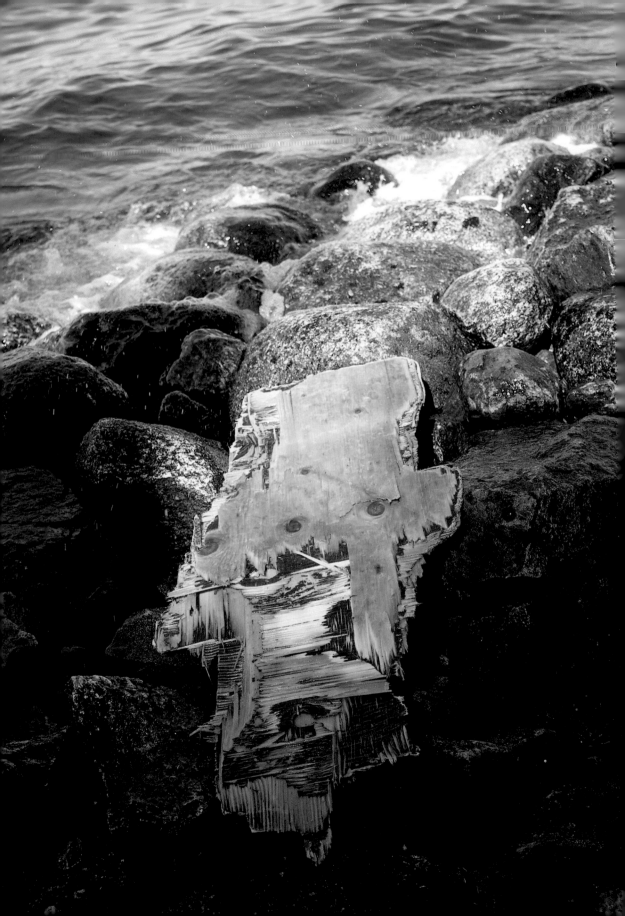

LCHQ Food Up Close

There are of course many types of foods that fit within the definition of LCHQ, but here is a list of my favorites with a description of why they are of such high quality.

🔲 **LEGUMES** contain high levels of protein and carbohydrates, and are very much worth their price. The number of carbs varies, but their glycemic index is always low. Since legumes do contain carbs, you can't eat them in large quantities when keeping to the LCHQ diet, but a reasonable amount is encouraged. Among legumes, there are lentils, peas, and beans—all of which are superfoods. They protect against many forms of cancer, cardiovascular disease, type 2 diabetes, and osteoporosis, and they also help maintain your weight. Colorful legumes, such as black beans and lentils or kidney beans, contain a significant amount of nutrients. There has been speculation about whether or not the phytoestrogen in soybeans could have a negative effect on male fertility but new research shows that this concern is unfounded (48).

All legumes contain something called lectin, which is a type of protein that exists naturally in beans, lentils, and peas, and inhibits the breakdown of starch. This is a good thing, because it contributes to a lower glycemic index. However, it can also cause negative effects, so it's important to maintain a balance. The main idea is to refrain from eating enough legumes to cause gas, diarrhea, or an upset stomach, since these conditions indicate you have had too much. Lectins will deactivate as a result of too much heat, so proper cooking is important. Generally, lentils and peas contain lower levels of lectin than beans, and the canned option is better than the dried ones, since drying implies that the container itself has been exposed to heat.

🔲 **MOLLUSKS** such as octopuses, mussels, and oysters are delicious protein bombs and are one of man's original food sources. One of my true favorites is the green-lipped mussel from the freezer aisle. It's generally pretty large, and the meat sticks to the shell. Plus, the meat contains the highly anti-inflammatory omega-3 fatty acid ETA.

🔲 **BOUILLON** is a great way to season your food without adding unnecessary calories. You can add a cube or a small piece to boiling rice, quinoa, meat sauce, and so on. It will provide a lot of flavor. Make sure you don't choose those that contain trans fats or flavor enhancers.

🔲 **BERRIES** are an extremely good source of antioxidants, regardless of whether they are frozen, fresh, or dried. In principle, all nutrients remain when the berries are frozen and are concentrated when they are dried. Watch out for sweetened berries, since they will take you above the carbohydrate limit. Berry powder is also a great way to enrich food with antioxidants, and can be found in various forms in the health food store.

🔲 **FISH** is a staple for all LCHQ menus. Regardless of which type you choose, the protein in fish will do wonders. They fill you up more per calorie when compared to other proteins and will reduce your blood pressure while simultaneously improving your sensitivity to insulin. Many people eat too little fish because they simply don't think they know how to prepare it. First of all, it's way simpler to cook fish than most people believe. The easiest way is to prepare a fish soup based on fish stock and vegetables; just remove it from the liquid from the stove and add pieces of raw salmon and white fish. The fish doesn't necessarily have to boil in order to be cooked, and this technique makes for a delicious soup. Secondly, there are several practical solutions to turn to: smoked or cured fish, vacuum sealed fish, canned tuna, mackerel, and sardines, as well as pickled herring. Sure, some of these alternatives contain small amounts of sugar, but it's insignificant and the benefits are infinitely greater than any negative effect.

There's also the opportunity of safely eating raw fish in the form of sushi and sashimi.

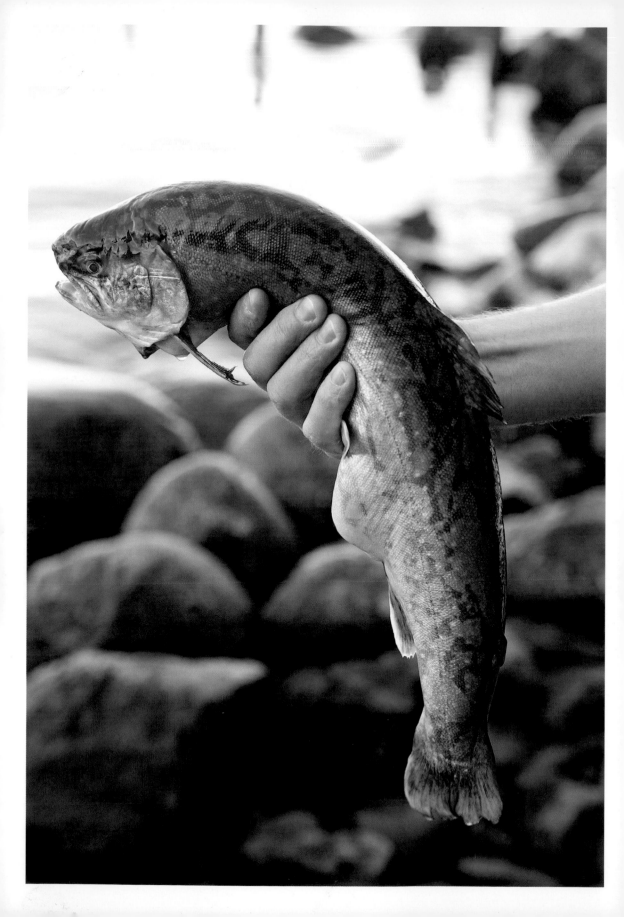

Additionally, raw Salma salmon is currently marketed as free from parasites, meaning it doesn't need to be frozen and can be eaten straight from the package. It's perfect for ad hoc sashimi.

I don't think you need to be intimidated by the thought of cooking fresh fish either—such as tuna, halibut, or cod.

Frozen fish is also fantastic. When fatty fish is frozen, a vacuum is usually created or the packaging is infused with nitrogen. This minimizes the oxygen, keeping the fish from going rancid and prolonging its shelf life. Nowadays, the grocery store stocks bags of frozen fish pieces, which is perfect for storing in the freezer for those days when you want to make a soup or stir fry.

🔍 **STOCKS** are great for casseroles, soups, etc. The nutrition labels often provide more clarity than those of bouillon cubes, and it's easy to find meat and vegetable stocks without flavor enhancers.

🔍 **FRUIT.** There are some people who claim that you can get fat from fruit. I argue that this is completely unfounded. Studies show that those who eat fruit every day are thinner than others (49, 50, 51)—fruit is one of the leanest types of foods there are. Only about 10 percent of a piece of fruit consists of carbohydrates. So a pear with 100 grams of "flesh" contains approximately 11 percent (11 grams) of carbs. Keeping in mind that the 20 percent from carbs the LCHQ diet calls for allows for 125 grams of carbs, this means that if you expend 2,500 calories per day, there is a whole lot of room for fruit snacking—as long as you keep your intake of carbs from other sources low. Once you've weaned yourself off of refined sugar, the sweetness of the fruit will become a real enjoyment and you can eat your favorite fruits every day guilt-free.

One trick is to cut the fruit into small bites and arrange them on a plate; this will make it feel a little more fancy than eating an apple straight up. Fruit contains more nutrients than just carbs. For example, pineapple and papaya contain enzymes that help your body break down protein. A small fruit salad with these fruits as a basis will therefore help your digestive system.

🔍 **SEEDS** are a real superfood when it comes to nutrients and the glycemic index. First of all, they make for a cocktail of healthy nutrients, such as fats, antioxidants, protein, vitamins, minerals, and extremely slow-acting carbohydrates—if any at all. Secondly, they delay the gastric emptying, so that the food and blood sugar is released into the body more slowly. This is why seeds have a natural glycemic index-reducing effect. Whether you choose flaxseed, pumpkin seeds, sunflower seeds, or psyllium seeds makes no difference—they're all great for you. However, the smallest seeds, such as flaxseed and sesame seeds, should be crushed before consumption in order for you to access their nutrients.

🔍 **POULTRY.** Chicken is the most common form of poultry in the grocery store, but don't forget about goose, turkey, ostrich, and duck—all of which have great nutritional value. High amounts of protein combined with a relatively low fat content makes these appropriate for LCHQ, as long as you don't forget to add fat from other sources as well. My personal favorite is the chicken thigh fillet, which is much more delicious than the chicken breast.

One advantage of poultry is that it contains less iron than red meat and is therefore less inflammatory. Red meat is only preferably if you suffer from an iron deficiency, and then wild meat and game is always the best option.

🔍 **GRAIN.** Oatmeal, rye flakes, and barleycorn are all rich in carbohydrates, so there's little room for them in the LCHQ diet. However, when you need carbs, these are a great solution. They contain many antioxidants and seem to protect against type 2 diabetes, some forms of cancer, and cardiovascular disease. The more intact the grain's structure, the more filling it will be, so it might be best to choose whole grain oats, whole grain wheat, or pearl barley.

🔍 **VEGETABLES.** If a food group is to be awarded the title of "best food in the universe," chances are good it will be vegetables. They're beautiful, delicious, and versatile. There are so few dishes in which vegetables don't have a place, either as an ingredient or a garnish. Vegetables are also often worth their price and are environmentally friendly. The list of their health benefits is long. Vegetables reduce blood pressure and expand the blood vessels, are anti-inflammatory, reduce blood fat, and are good for your weight. They also increase insulin sensitivity and reduce the risk of many types of cancer, and they enable your brain to thrive. Vegetables also help the stomach by providing it with the right type of (water-soluble) fibers.

If your stomach is sensitive to raw vegetables, you can cook them. This not only makes them easier to digest, but also helps you absorb the nutrients better. Antioxidants are often easier to absorb if you cook the vegetables—the process of which will also be improved if you add fat. There are, of course, hundreds—if not thousands—of vegetables from around the world to choose from, but these are some of my favorites in terms of flavor and nutritional value: eggplant, squash, bell pepper, tomato (crushed, sundried, purée), avocado, corn, all types of lettuce, broccoli and other types of cabbage, asparagus, Jerusalem artichoke, artichoke, and sprouts of all kinds. Onions, such as yellow and red, chives, garlic, scallions, and leeks contain sulfurous substances that are very nutritious and will boost your body's own production of antioxidants.

HONEY naturally contains a lot of carbohydrates, but in small amounts it is perfectly all right in the LCHQ diet. Studies have found that honey not only keeps us thin, but also provides a healthy supplement of antioxidants. Despite honey's sweetness, it has a low glycemic index. It's also antibacterial and antiviral, which contributes to the soothing effect of honey-infused water. Make sure you don't heat honey too much; the health benefits of honey decrease if it's exposed to temperatures above 150°F (65°C). It doesn't matter whether you choose liquid, solid, light, or dark honey, but more color means more antioxidants. Liquid honey contains more fructose than its solid equivalent, but otherwise they are similar.

COCONUT. The coconut isn't really a nut. It's actually a seed. which makes it edible for most people with nut allergies. Coconut oil consists of 60 to 70 percent short and medium saturated fats. These are more water-soluble than long-chain fatty acids, which are stored in your fat cells. Therefore, coconut oil doesn't have the same ability to be stored as fat and is instead directly used to fuel the liver and the muscles. This causes an increased energy expenditure in the liver and increased amounts of energy your muscles can use. The latter provides you with more stamina and a desire to exercise and move. One thing that contributes to the workout benefits of eating short and medium saturated fats is that they can be sent directly to your muscles' powerhouses. These are called the mitochondria and they serve to transform what you eat into a running stride or other forms of movement. Long-chain fats take longer to reach the mitochondria, since they require carnitine in order to be transported in. The medium and short-chain fats do not require carnitine and can therefore be burnt off much more quickly. Coconut oil also has a tendency to fill us up more than other fats. For example, don't you find that a Thai curry can be really filling? One reason is because of the short- and medium-chain fats' ability to be used directly in the liver, and when the body spends them, the liver's temperature rises. A higher temperature reduces your appetite, which is something you've probably noticed during the summertime or while on vacation in a warm country. You simply don't eat as much at these times, which makes it easier to maintain your weight.

One significant detail is that coconut oil contains about 5 percent fewer calories than other sources of fat, which can have a huge impact if you eat coconut oil on a daily basis. This is due to the high quantity of medium- and short-chain fatty acids, which naturally contain a lower calorie content. But just as with most fat, coconut oil can generate an energy surplus, which can cause weight gain. It's just more difficult for this to occur with coconut oil than with other fats.

Another benefit is that the lauric acid found in coconut oil has antibacterial characteristics and can also be converted into monolaurin—a fatty acid with an very strong antibacterial effect.

This can contribute to a better intestinal flora, better long-term gastrocolic health, and a stronger immune system. Research has also found that monolaurin can prevent yeast infections and protect against various intestinal parasites. Some studies have shown that it may protect against hepatitis, influenza, and the measles. A high level of lauric acid has also been shown to decrease the risk for depression, which sounds logical since the brain consists of fat. Thus, the quality of the fat will certainly affect brain functionality.

A fresh coconut contains approximately 33 percent fat, of which 90 percent is saturated. The coconut's 9 percent fiber content is considered very high and the glycemic index is low. The 3.3 percent protein content is higher than in fruit, and coconuts specifically contain zinc, potassium, phosphorus, magnesium, iron, vitamin B6, and folic acid. It has also been claimed that coconut can increase the uptake of vitamins and minerals from other types of foods.

SPICES are a concentrate of antioxidants and lots of other exciting nutrients. Quite simply, almost all spices cause some form of health benefit. Saffron can stimulate the immune system (52), and black pepper and turmeric appear to serve as antidepressants, since they increase the level of serotonin in the brain (53, 54). Mustard appears to inhibit the growth of cancerous tumors (55), and ginger is highly anti-inflammatory (56). Wasabi has shown to protect against osteoporosis; cinnamon is known for balancing blood sugar levels so effectively that it's a natural aid for type 2 diabetes (58). Curry exists in myriad forms—the common denominator of which is their high levels of antioxidants, which seem to prevent dementia and the decrease of mental capacity in the elderly (59).

The list of spices with positive health benefits can go on and on. Therefore, you should really use spices over artificial flavors, scents, and flavor enhancers. Since LCHQ relies on real food with many spices, you will receive that high-quality effect even here.

MEAT is also allowed in the LCHQ diet, for those who choose to eat it. Red meat is rich in protein, iron, vitamin B14, and other healthy substances, but unfortunately, the modern meat we are used to purchasing is not really that healthy. This is because livestock are fed carbohydrate-rich grain products that create long-chained saturated fats in the animals' bodies. Additionally, the meat from cattle is too fatty. Wild animals are constantly in movement and are fit, which generates a leaner meat with unsaturated fat and even omega-3s. Research has found that beef from cattle increases inflammation, while game meat does not (10). Therefore, there is plenty of research that indicates that it's not the meat itself that increases the risk for cardiovascular disease, cancer, and obesity, but the modern-day fat constellation that the meat contains (11). Plus, game is also preferable when it comes to ethical issues, and it causes less environmental waste than meat from livestock.

Air-dried game makes for a great snack and contains almost double the amount of protein as fresh meat. Ground game meat is also excellent. If one of your friends enjoys hunting, see if he/she will share some of the catch with you.

MAYONNAISE. Homemade mayonnaise is, of course, preferable to store bought, since you'll only use natural ingredients. If you want to try making your own homemade mayonnaise, there are many great recipes online and in cookbooks. Even commercially available mayonnaise is fine to eat as long as it's made with canola oil. Sure, it contains additives, but that's not a particularly big problem, since they're usually the more harmless types. You also should not eat high quantities of it.

DAIRY PRODUCTS are often great sources of protein. For example, hard cheese contains about 30 percent protein, beating out meat, poultry, and fish. Yogurt is also excellent, since it contains lactic acid bacteria that are good for your stomach and immune system. Cottage cheese and quark are high-quality, protein-rich, and low-fat foods that make tasty snacks. Adding cottage cheese to yogurt is a quick and inexpensive way of increasing the protein content in the food. Some yogurts contain a little more fat, but these are usually a good base for sauces and tzatziki. It also appears that dairy fat is better than we originally thought, for both your heart and overall fitness. This is due to the fact that dairy fat contains short and medium saturated fats, with a high content of monounsaturated omega 9 fat.

In general, it's a good idea to choose lean dairy products, as long as you get fats from other healthy sources. It is, of course, very easy to get enormous amounts of calories from crème fraiche and heavy cream.

NUTS are some of the best things you can eat. They lower the glycemic index of the foods you eat them with, and they provide a lot of nutrients: healthy fats, proteins, fibers, antioxidants, vitamins, and minerals, as well as trace amounts of carbohydrates. It's difficult to say which nuts are the healthiest, since they all have their benefits. Cashews, hazelnuts, macadamia nuts, and almonds all contain high levels of antioxidants, most of which you will find in those with the darkest inner shell. Walnuts are unique because of their high omega-3 content, whereas pecans actually win the antioxidant contest.

A very interesting study found that the anti-inflammatory capacity is actually higher in roasted nuts, as opposed to natural nuts (60). It's unclear if this is true for all nuts, but it might not be a bad idea to choose the most delicious roasted nuts you can find for a snack, instead of chips, cheese doodles, and the like.

Brazil nuts are interesting because they contain a lot of selenium, of which many people suffer a deficiency. Selenium is important because it's used in the body's production of antioxidants, and a deficiency will increase the risk for cardiovascular disease and cancer. Research has found that it's enough to eat just two Brazil nuts a day to cause a significant increase in the body's levels of selenium and production of the body's own antioxidant, called glutathione peroxidase, in the blood (62).

OLIVE OIL is what I personally use for just about everything I cook. It's both delicious and contains better quality fat than most other oils. With 70 to 80 percent monounsaturated fat, it's great for the heart, protects against type 2 diabetes, and helps us maintain our weight. In fact, it's not only the monounsaturated fat in the olive oil that protects against cardiovascular disease (61) but also something else that we think is the polyphenol oleocanthal (antioxidant). This apparently has very strong anti-inflammatory characteristics and is even chemically related to ibuprofen (63). Oleocanthal provides olive oil with its bitter, peppery flavor, and the more flavor, the more likely it is that the oil contains high levels of the oleocanthal. It should also protect against inflammation in other parts of the body. Since autoimmune diseases, type 2 diabetes, and other painful things are caused by inflammation, olive oil is highly interesting.

Olive oil has also been found to protect against breast and colon cancer, probably due to the fact that it contains squalene, which is a relative of human cholesterol. Olive oil also contains the powerful antioxidants tyrosol and hydroxytyrosol, both of which are antibacterial and can prevent gastrointestinal infections. Naturally, olives themselves are also very healthy and provide the body with such substances as fibers.

PROTEIN POWDER is a protein concentrate that is very useful—despite being a powder. If you're thinking about buying protein powder, you should ensure that it's clean—that is to say, free from fat, carbohydrates, and other additives such as sweeteners or scents. Many powders contain high levels of carbs, which generates an undesirable blood sugar response and violates the limit of 20 E% from carbohydrates within the LCHQ diet.

Carbs found in protein powder are rarely healthy, since they usually derive from refined sugars such as fructose or glucose, or highly glycemic forms of starch like maltodextrin. My advice is to refrain from overusing protein powder since there's a risk of your developing lactose intolerance. In one portion containing 35 grams of protein, you receive as many carbs as in a quart of milk, so a couple of servings of protein powder every day provides

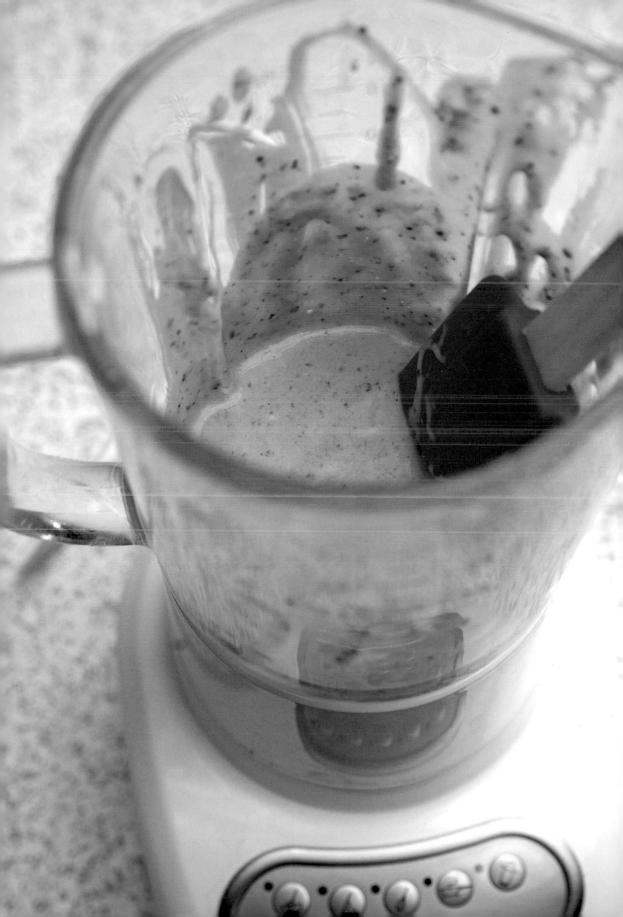

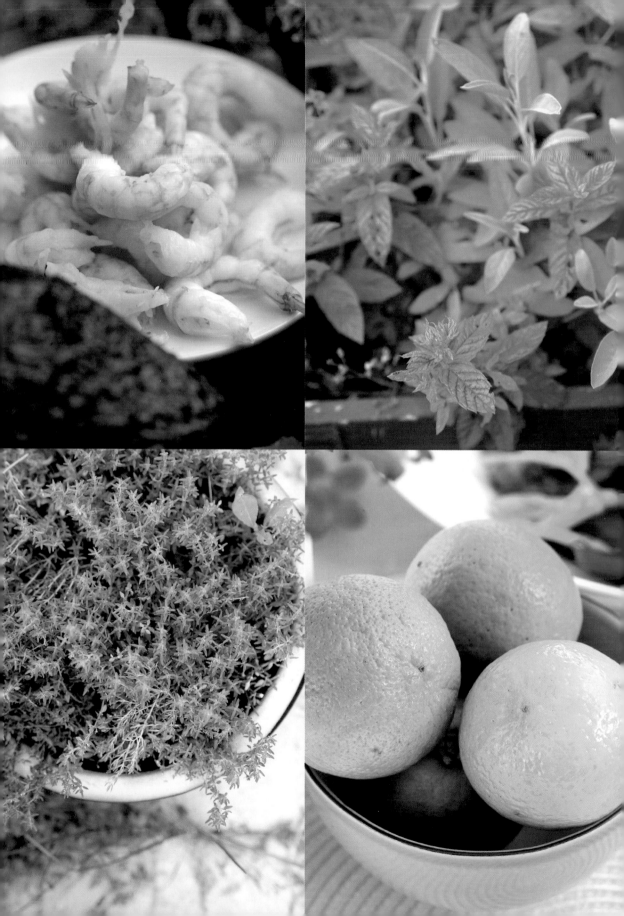

an unnaturally high intake of proteins from a single source.

Protein powder is especially appropriate for the first post-workout meal (perhaps along with an apple). It will provide a speedy recovery at a point when your muscles are most receptive. Milk protein is equally great, as well as whey and casein. The latter two are a natural part of milk protein, but can also be found concentrated as protein powder. Soy protein is great for people who are lactose intolerant or need some variety.

An important thing to keep in mind is that protein powder isn't a natural product, which LCHQ requires, so I completely understand that one may wish to exclude it.

Q **QUINOA** is one of my favorites in the carbohydrate category. It's delicious and healthy, with a low glycemic index, and it's rich in protein, fibers, and antioxidants. Quinoa is actually a natural whole grain product, since nothing has been refined or removed from the original seed. I like to cook a little extra quinoa to sprinkle on top of my salad the next day.

Q **CANOLA OIL** contains the omega 3 fatty acid ALA, which can be converted to DHA in the body. In other words, it's the same fatty acid that exists in fish. There are also many monounsaturated and polyunsaturated fats in the form of linoleic acid in canola oil. This makes canola oil better for cardiovascular health than such things as dairy fat, for example (65). The healthiest type is cold pressed canola oil, but even the refined option has great health benefits. It has a distinctive taste that doesn't fit all recipes, but the colorless variety is usually all right.

Q **RICE** is also a great source of carbs. Even if the LCHQ diet doesn't leave much room for it, brown rice is one of the best things with which to fill your carb quota. It exists in different colors, including black, red, and brown. Regardless of which one you choose, it will have a low glycemic index and high nutritional value.

Q **ROOT VEGETABLES** are God's gift to LCHQ proponents! Carrots, beets, parsnips, and rutabagas provide a lot of food but few carbohydrates: 8.7 percent for carrots; 8.5 percent for beets; 10.2 percent for parsnips; and 6.4 percent for rutabagas. If you want to try a really low-carb dish with root vegetables, you should cook LCHQ root vegetables with salmon and feta (see page 84) in which we use root vegetables with the fewest carbs. You can eat potatoes with LCHQ, but since LCHQ allows for only a small amount, it's wiser to choose other root vegetables. After all, a boiled and peeled potato contains 19 percent carbohydrates.

Q **SALT** is needed for flavor and is completely harmless to most people. However, some people with high blood pressure react positively to lowering their salt intake. Usually we refer to these people as "salt sensitive," but most people with abnormally high blood pressure usually get better results through other means. A higher consumption of potassium and magnesium lowers blood pressure, as does lower glycemic pressure, healthy fats, and regular exercise. This is all provided with the LCHQ diet, so I don't believe that the salt is worrisome.

If you're sensitive to salt, you can use mineral salt, which consists mostly of potassium chloride as opposed to sodium chloride (which is what regular salt consists of). Personally, I use sea salt for most things. The main reason for this is that it contains trace elements from the ocean that are healthy for our bodies—even if these benefits are difficult to study due to the microscopic amounts that we consume.

Furthermore, I think that sea salt tastes better because of its more "rounded" taste as opposed to the more "acrid" character of regular table salt. If you do use table salt, the kinds with added iodine are best, since this contributes to your body's production of thyroid hormones.

Q **SHELLFISH** doesn't have to be as expensive as you might think. You can often find frozen, unpeeled shrimp at bargain prices in the grocery store, and the smaller the size, the cheaper they are. Crayfish tails are also worth the cost, and crab is a great seasonal delicacy in the early fall. Lobster is, of course, one of the more expensive varieties.

Regardless of which kind of shellfish you choose, they're all very healthy. The protein content is high and the little fat they contain is of high quality. Their pink color stems from the antioxidant Astaxanthin, which is a healthy carotenoid that protects your cells. One of my favorite LCHQ meals is a small shellfish platter with homemade aioli and a glass of red wine. It's the perfect dish for the end of the day, since it contains very few carbohydrates.

FOOD FLAVORINGS give a dish one or more extra layers. Food should be delicious and make you feel great. Pleasure generates reward chemicals in the brain, which makes you appreciate life more. Great examples are pesto and tapenade, which both contain a lot of calories, but only from good ingredients. Capers are one of my favorites for salads and other things, and they're practically calorie-free and can be used without restraint. Tabasco is another example of a great flavoring that is not only calorie-free, but also increases your energy expenditure, so you can more easily maintain your weight. Fish sauce and soy sauce are very high in sodium, but provide lots of extra flavor because they are fermented products. They fit great within LCHQ.

GRAINS appear in very low quantities in LCHQ. Whole grain oats, bulgur, whole grain wheat, pearl barley, buckwheat, oatmeal, rye flakes, etc. are all great products but contain high amounts of carbohydrates, which limits their usability. If you keep the LCHQ diet but exercise a lot and want to increase your intake of carbs, these are the ingredients you should eat more of.

MUSHROOMS are great LCHQ ingredients. Portobellos, chanterelles, morels, and shiitake mushrooms are my personal favorites. They don't contain a lot of energy, but they provide fibers, minerals, and trace elements, as well as some very distinct flavors to improve your meal.

SAUCES with a high calorie content, such as béarnaise sauce, hollandaise sauce, and remoulade, should be consumed in moderation

and, if possible, should be made from scratch. This will help you avoid the high amount of additives in commercial sauces, and you can choose the best oil for the cooking. Tzatziki and feta cheese scramble are great examples of sauces that provide the creamy feel without consisting of about 100 E% fat.

TOFU is a special product that fits well within the concept of LCHQ. It consists of about 2 percent carbohydrates, 5 percent fat, and 8 percent protein, so a salad with a large piece of tofu is great. Tofu can also be used in casseroles, smoothies, and so on. Your imagination is the limit, but note that as a vegan it's almost impossible to eat LCHQ without including tofu.

VINEGAR is sour, and sour foods reduce the glycemic index of the food you consume. Vinegar is therefore great in salads, sauces, or perhaps for making pickled salmon. It also enhances flavors. Preferably choose red wine vinegar, since it contains the highest amount of antioxidants.

EGGS are a fantastically complete food. One egg contains approximately 7 grams of protein, of which 4 grams reside in the yolk. The egg yolk also contains an incredible amount of vitamins, minerals, and antioxidants. If you choose omega-3 eggs, the quality of the fat is almost perfect. It's simply a food staple.

HERBS have a plethora of almost magical characteristics. Regardless of whether they are fresh or dry, they're probably the single most beneficial type of food for your health.

"If a food group is to be awarded the title of 'best food in the universe,' chances are good it will be vegetables."

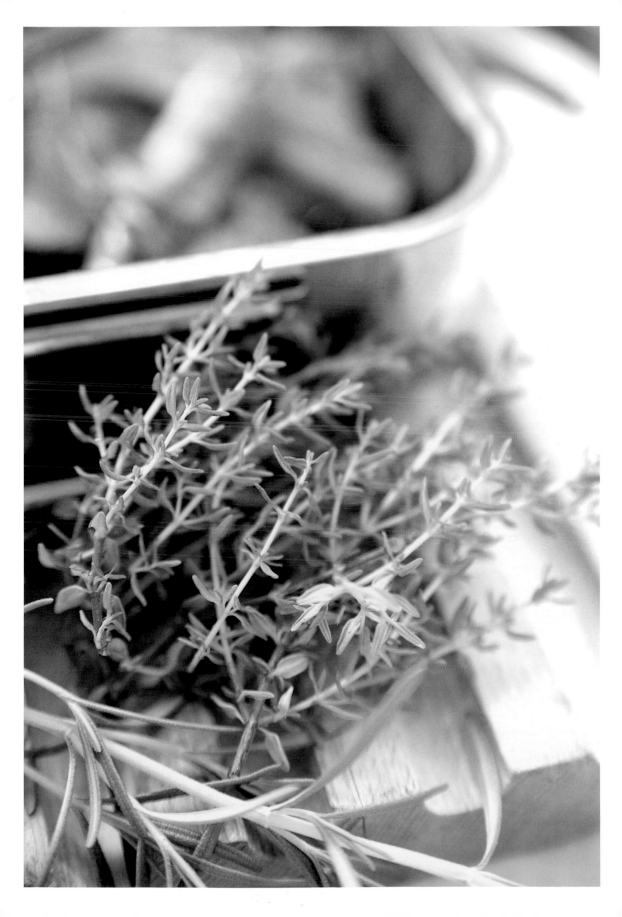

Beverages and LCHQ

Some beverages can make you fat and sick, while others may keep you thin and healthy. The main idea is to avoid beverages with added sugar. I'm sure you know most of them: lemonade, soda, sweetened juices, alcohol. Soda is particularly common in our culture, and just one a day can increase the risk for type 2 diabetes. Since many people drink soda by the liter, this becomes a huge public health issue. Diet soda is not a good alternative, since it increases appetite, especially for sweet things.

If you want a sweet beverage, you should drink fruit juice—just be sure you're not accidentally drinking a high-in-sugar fruit drink. Admittedly, juices contain some carbohydrates, but they're also filled with antioxidants, vitamins, minerals, and even fibers. Pulp actually consists of fibers. Therefore, real juice is a healthy alternative to sugary beverages, but you should drink them in moderation if you want to keep the LCHQ diet. For example, if you eat a meal of chicken drumsticks and vegetable juice, totaling about five hundred calories, a hundred of those should come from the juice. This translates to about 8.5 oz (250 ml) of juice and 10 percent carbohydrates. In this case, juice is a great beverage, especially if it contains high levels of antioxidants! If the food is complete in all other regards in terms of nutrients, water is the best alternative, regardless of whether or not it's carbonated, as long as it's not sweetened. Tea, coffee, and red wine have their functions, but they deserve their own separate section.

disease. The tea leaves themselves actually contain more caffeine per gram than coffee does, but since less tea is used per cup than the equivalent in coffee, the level of caffeine is about 30–90 milligrams per 250 milliliters. Coffee contains about two or three times that amount. All sorts of teas are allowed in LCHQ, but remember to factor in the honey that you use when counting your daily ration of carbs.

Coffee is also rich in antioxidants and a myriad other great substances—we have identified about a thousand so far. There are many health benefits and research has found that it protects against type 2 diabetes, depression, gout, cirrhosis, Parkinson's disease, and Alzheimer's, as well as cardiovascular disease. Of course, coffee also fits in the LCHQ diet, since it is free from calories and can be consumed in relatively large quantities without any proven negative heath effects.

Caffeine in tea and coffee is known for providing energy, and also for releasing dopamine in the brain. Since dopamine is a reward chemical that makes us feel good, coffee and tea drinkers generally consider their quality of life to be higher than those who exclude these beverages. As a result, they are very much a part of the LCHQ concept. Adding sugar to one's coffee is of course a big no-no, since the amount of sugar you consume if you drink a lot of coffee adds up quickly.

Tea and coffee improves quality further

One particularly good type of tea is brewed from the *Camellia sinensis* plant and contains many interesting substances, such as caffeine, theanine, and antioxidants. Up to 30 percent of the fresh leaf's dry weight can consist of catechins—highly potent antioxidants that appear to inhibit the development of cancer and decrease the risk for cardiovascular

Reasonable amounts of alcohol are allowed

Alcohol is actually one of the energy providing nutrients, but not something that is absolutely necessary for survival. Lots of research shows that alcohol—mostly in terms of red wine—actually has a positive effect on your health and weight. It seems impossible that a "poison" like alcohol could provide better cardiovascular health and reduced risk of type 2 diabetes and weight loss. However, you should take into account that we're talking about a maximum of one or two glasses of red wine per day, and that it's particularly red wine (not white or blush) that is beneficial. Through red wine, you can receive not only the alcohol but also many antioxidants. If you have difficulty stopping before you drink too much, it's better to exclude alcohol completely—especially as it's an addictive substance. If you drink too much, it definitely causes more harm than good; it puts pressure on your heart, liver, kidneys, brain, and pancreas—your entire body, really. A surplus of alcohol also increases blood pressure, stores fat, and increases the risk for cancer. It may be superfluous to mention that an abuse of alcohol also clouds your judgment; however, a moderate intake of red wine is great for the LCHQ diet.

Even if alcohol provides energy, you don't have to include it in your calorie count. As you remember, LCHQ allows for 20 E% carbohydrates, 40 E% from protein, and the same amount from fat. Maintain these ratios between fat, protein, and carbohydrates as before, and make sure red wine is only an occasional enjoyment in your everyday life.

Why only red wine?

Of course it's okay to have the occasional glass of white wine, beer, or champagne. But regular consumption of alcohol should, if anything, consist of red wine only. Red wine is the most beneficial for your health as it contributes much more than just the alcohol.

Here's a quick run-through of the advantages of red wine over other alcoholic beverages.

Red wine contains both melatonin and resveratrol, two substances that appear to protect against cardiovascular disease (12).

Red wine does not increase the risk of osteoporosis in the same way as pure alcohol, and perhaps it could even provide a certain protection thereof (13).

Red wine reduces the uptake of oxidized (rancid) cholesterol after your meal (14). In the study cited, you can see that a double cheeseburger increases the amount of oxidized cholesterol in the blood, and red wine virtually eliminated the problem.

Since oxidized cholesterol gets stuck in the blood vessels, it might explain why red wine reduces the risk of cardiovascular disease.

While other sources of alcohol seem to increase the risk of certain types of cancer, red wine has been found to not be as bad. In fact, red wine has been shown to reduce the risk of, for example, bladder cancer (15).

The resveratrol in red wine expands the blood vessels, which contributes to a lower blood pressure and risk of cardiovascular disease (16). Resveratrol is also anti-inflammatory and strengthens the immune system. It has also been found to inhibit ageing in test animals (17).

Red wine has been found to have a positive impact on the immune system. One or two glasses each day could reduce the risk of a cold and other infections (28).

The HQ in LCHQ

As you may recall, HQ is an abbreviation for High Quality, referring not only to the nutrients but also to the quality of life. Therefore, red wine's inclusion in the LCHQ diet is very positive. Dinner will be more enjoyable, and food will taste better with a nice pairing of red wine. LCHQ is a lifestyle, and life's too short to live ascetically, without any enjoyment. But the pleasure should focus on long-term well-being, which is the role of red wine.

When you drink red wine, your brain's reward system is activated, similar to when fat and sugar are consumed. When you receive the reward of a glass of wine, your craving for fat and sugar is reduced and it is be easier to resist dessert or candy.

This way, it might be easier to maintain fitness.

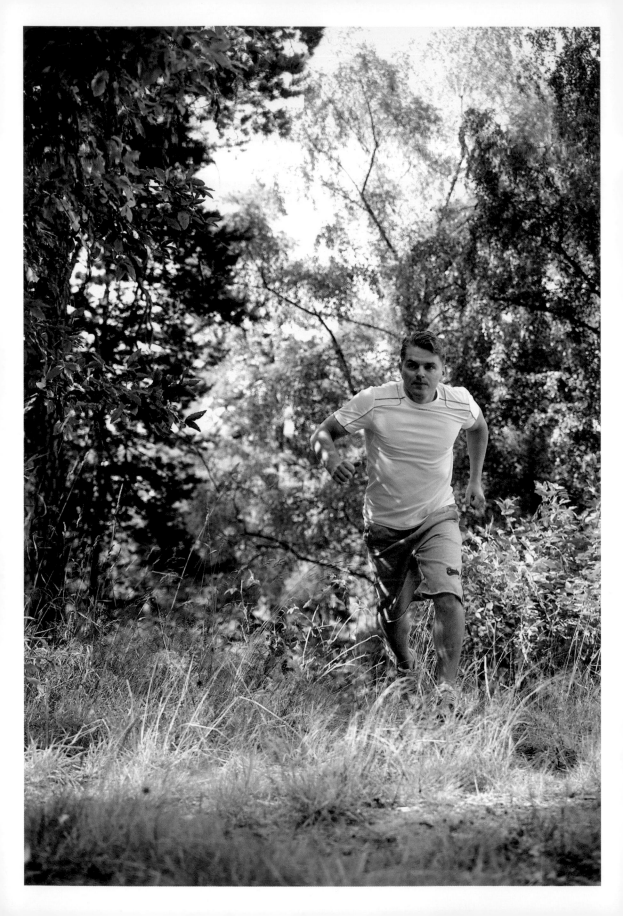

Exercise

LCHQ is, as you know, not a pure weight loss diet, but it keeps body fat low with much more ease. The reason why you burn more fat is the distribution between the nutrients. It's actually very simple: You burn what you eat, and if you eat more carbohydrates, you will burn off carbohydrates.

It will also give you more energy for exercise, but the best thing is you burn both carbs and fat at the same time. This is how you get the most out of your muscles, and this enables you to handle both aerobic and anaerobic exercise.

Aerobic exercise means that you exercise at a low or medium intensity, such as by walking or jogging. Even aerobics and cardio machines have many anaerobic parts and you can generally say that the higher the intensity, the more anaerobic your exercise is.

The harder you work, the more carbs you will expend, and with extreme, purely anaerobic exercise—such as weightlifting—you will almost exclusively use carbs as fuel. Endurance training still works fine on a low-carb diet but as soon as you want to achieve anaerobic capacity, your must include at least some carbohydrates in your diet.

If you follow a carbohydrate-based diet, as many athletes used to and to an extent still do, the amount of carbs you expend will be greater. When carbohydrates are used, lactic acid will develop and we all know how that feels in our muscles. This means that a high-carb diet may actually worsen your endurance, whereas an extreme low-carb diet decreases strength and anaerobic capacity. LCHQ is the perfect middle ground.

When you follow LCHQ, you will notice a couple of things. Since the carbohydrate intake is low, your body will be forced to use more fat as fuel, which will increase your fat expenditure. The relatively high intake of protein further increases your fat expenditure and if you're used to exercising, this will manifest itself in the form of shortness of breath. It's not that you lose your breath more, since you definitely have enough energy, but it's because the fat requires approximately 10 percent more oxygen than carbs when it's being used. This means you need 10 percent more breaths in order to supply your muscles with enough oxygen.

Exercising = good health

If you really want to achieve super health, it's not enough to simply eat well; regular physical activity is also necessary. Exercise has been found to protect against a plethora of diseases and reduce the discomfort of equally as many. We know that regular exercise reduces the risk of cancer, cardiovascular disease, type 2 diabetes, depression, osteoporosis, high blood pressure, inflammations, autoimmune diseases, infections, and of course obesity. In some cases, the mechanisms are clearly demonstrated. For example, we know that exercising stimulates the production of endorphins, serotonin, and dopamine, which makes people with an active lifestyle enjoy better mental health. In terms of on obesity, it is pretty self-evident that increased energy expenditure helps reduce the body's fat repositories.

But you cannot always explain the whole effect. Today, some are talking about an "exercise factor," in other words something unknown that contributes to the positive effects of exercise (43). Some scientists claim that it has to do with so-called myokines, a type of peptide that is released from fit muscles (44). These peptides behave like a hormone (without actually being one) and could be the reason for everything from increased muscle and tissue to lower blood pressure and a strengthened immune system. Hopefully, research will clarify the full effect of myokines and perhaps generate new ways of exercising.

Learn from my mistakes

My philosophy is: "Don't exercise hard, exercise smart." This means, don't work out so intensely that you risk incurring a brain bleed or for so long that your joints get worn down and inflamed. Personally, I used to exercise way too hard and too early. When I was in my twenties, I could easily work out twice a day. In the morning, I would lift weights, and in the evenings I would do martial arts. I would have a day of rest now and then, but it was much too little, and in combination with a poor diet, my joints got inflamed. Back in those days, at the end of the '80s and beginning of the '90s, fat was banned and carbs were celebrated for their performance-enhancing characteristics.

That was before we knew about the glycemic index and how fast-acting the carbohydrates were, so I stuffed myself with carbs and very little fat to align with that era's recommended diet. Since anti-inflammatory omega-3 fats were scarce in my diet and many of the carbs were of the fast-acting kind, my body was afflicted with constant inflammations.

Hard exercise and a pro-inflammatory diet seem to feed off each other, and my hands and feet started to hurt so badly that I had to take painkillers every day in order to make it out of bed in the morning. The shoulders are particularly at risk when you work out intensely, and in my case it led to impingement on both shoulder blades.

That means the shoulders are afflicted with inflammations that generate small bone spurs clinging to the shoulder blade tissue. This causes a chronic condition in which the space between the shoulder joints becomes too tight; in my case, this caused constant pain and inflammation. As a result, I was forced to have operations on both shoulders, and today I'm completely free from pain. But if I exercise too hard and don't follow a proper diet, I risk repeating the same condition.

My exercise today

To me, physical activity is a necessity. I only have one body and I owe it the best possible care. It doesn't matter how healthily you eat—if you don't exercise, you will not achieve optimum health. Having healthy exercising habits is a way of thought.

I know that my body needs to be exposed to something that gets my pulse pumping every now and then, preferably every day. But if I constantly work out in intervals of several hours, or try to beat my personal best in terms of time, repetitions, or weights, I will ultimately push myself too hard. Surely you could do this from time to time, but for most people it's trivial how quickly you run or how heavy you lift. Personally, I don't know exactly how far I jog, but I think it's about 2.5 miles (4 km) every time. The most important thing for me is that the track is inspiring; I have a favorite path that leads me alongside beautiful archipelago beaches where the water is constantly in sight.

In that environment it never becomes too difficult to run, even when I'm going uphill, and it's too hot, and my legs are still sore from last time. The environment is therefore very important, and is probably the reason why many people fail to use the expensive exercise bike in the living room.

When I was younger, it was important what the weights read, and when I exercised most, I used 110 lbs (50 kg) weights for bench pressing. That is a lot for a guy who weighs 165 lbs (75 kg). Today, the number of pounds I lift is completely uninteresting to me. I know the consequences of training too intensely and too often, and I would like to be able to exercise for the rest of my life. Therefore, I simply use the weights that feel good at the time, and it doesn't matter what the label reads.

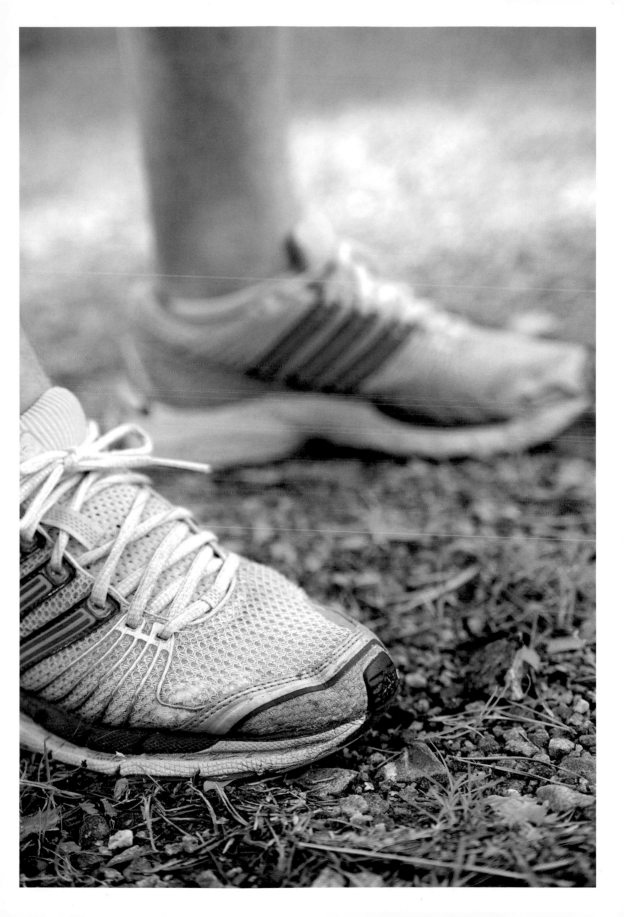

That is something to keep in mind when you start working out at the gym; feeling self-conscious about other toned members laughing at how weak you are. The truth is, no one cares if you use weights of 2.2 lbs (1 kg) or 44 lbs (20 kg). Everyone is busy with his or her own workout. You will get respect from your environment simply for going to the gym.

Today, my weightlifting workouts are rarely very long. They take about an hour in the gym, and when I exercise at home they usually take 30 minutes or I'll go for a jog for an equal length of time. I usually run every other day because otherwise I start to feel pain in my feet and knees. Days I don't run, I walk. Usually my whole family comes along but if not, I do a 60-minute power walk. It is more beneficial than you'd think!

Start slowly

I don't exercise nearly as much as I did before and I rarely work out for more than one hour. Many overly ambitious people decide to start a new life and create a workout schedule that would look familiar to elite athletes. It is very popular to sign up for various runs. Short ones are, of course, beneficial, especially if you do not suffer from any injuries and have the training for them. However, I have seen too many people focus on real challenges such as marathons and the like, who then suffer from injuries for a long time afterward. The groin, leg muscles, and calves suffer more than they can handle when you decide to run 26 miles (42 km).

Of course, there are people who can handle that type of stress, but most can't and they pay a high price for it physically. Research has shown that really intense exercise when you are not in good enough shape can harm the muscles of the heart. Therefore, you should start your workout endeavor slowly and build a solid foundation. You should also make sure to eat anti-inflammatory food, such as the LCHQ diet prescribes.

How to optimize your workouts

If you're used to exercising you will probably be fine on your own, and you can skip this section. If you're new to physical activity, the following section will be important. If you have some kind of disability or are obese and don't think my advice will work for you, you should adjust the suggestions to your own ability.

Essentially, I believe that a combination of three walks and three weight-lifting sessions per week is optimal for most people. The walks

POWER WALKS

Sure, it's nice to go for a relaxing walk without focusing on exercising, and it is indeed good for your well-being. But if you really want to maximize workout benefits, you ought to try power walking. It is not as tough as you might think, and it gets your pulse going while providing you with better exercising benefits than normal walks. I personally wear running shoes and workout clothes that are fit for sweating, because you will sweat.

The goal is to walk 10–20 percent quicker than usual and push each step a little more. That way, there is more pressure on your calves, buttocks, and thighs.

Preferably choose a path with a lot of hills since that generates a much better effect. When you encounter a hill, you should use the incline to push each step even more. Around one hour is great for power walks, but if you have more energy feel free to extend the walk. It is wise to stretch your muscles after a power walk as they have received more exercise than after a normal walk.

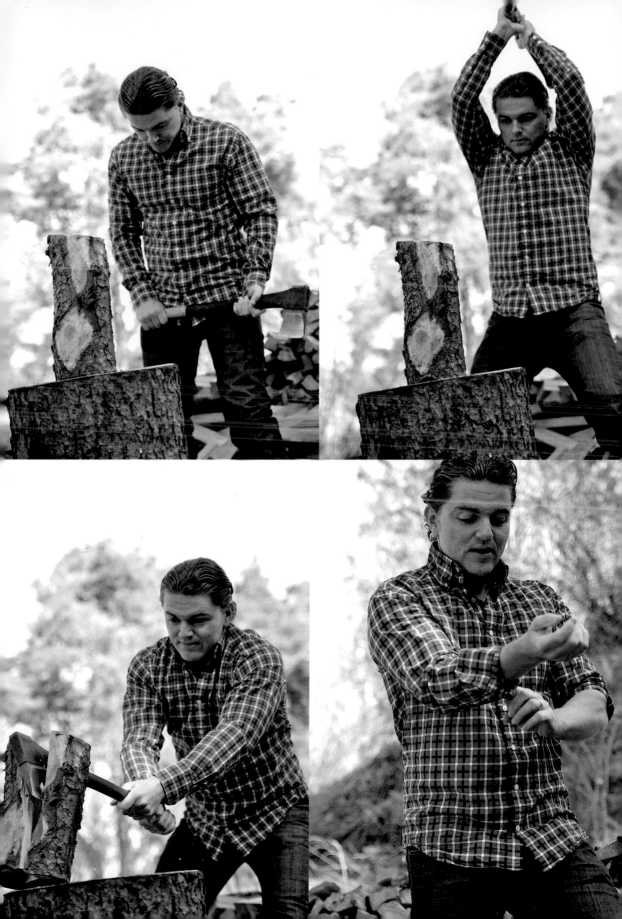

should last about 45–60 minutes, and can, of course, be replaced by other physical activities such as running, skiing, gardening, or another equivalent exercise for the same duration.

Weightlifting sessions can be very different. Circuit training—when you exercise all muscles in the same session—fits a lot of people since it is simple, fun, and doesn't require much knowledge. Another form of weightlifting is to divide up the different muscle groups so that you exercise each group once per week. This means dividing up the exercising of the chest, shoulders, upper back, lower back, biceps (front of arms), triceps (back of arms), front of thighs, back of thighs, buttocks, and calves.

It's good to work the abdominal muscles more frequently since they are important for reducing back pain and maintaining the ability to exercise. The best thing is, of course, to consult a personal trainer, especially when you are unfamiliar with the machines/equipment.

The best approach is to alternate between walking and weightlifting so that you dedicate yourself to both every other day. This reduces the risk of wear, injuries, and boredom. It also enables the body to recuperate from the workout it did the day before, which improves results. If you don't like gyms or there are none within a reasonable distance, you can also work out in your home. It is just as effective as the gym, but requires you to buy some equipment. You also need knowledge about how to use that equipment, which is something that home training books can provide you with.

Increase your everyday exercise

I think that the best exercise routine is the one described above but sometimes travel, vacation, sickness, and lack of motivation get in the way. Remind yourself that it's okay to devote yourself to alternative exercise. One method is to become more active in your everyday life, even if it takes fighting off some of your inherent laziness. A pedometer is a good way of doing so. Today there are some very advanced pedometers that create personalized goals for you and make a daily evaluation of whether or not you achieved them. If you see that you're a couple miles short, it is easy to motivate yourself to take an extra walk with the dog or to put in a couple of minutes on the treadmill.

Many have written about everyday exercise, but they often fail to take individual ability into consideration. When it comes to everyday exercise, you are your own personal trainer. When there is no opportunity for regular exercise, try to make your life a little more physically taxing. For example, take the stairs instead of the elevator or get off the bus one stop earlier. I really want to push for doing this in combination with having a smart pedometer. Then, you get a receipt for how much you're getting for your everyday exercise.

"It is good to alternate between walking and weightlifting so that you dedicate yourself to both every other day. This reduces the risk of wear, injuries, and boredom."

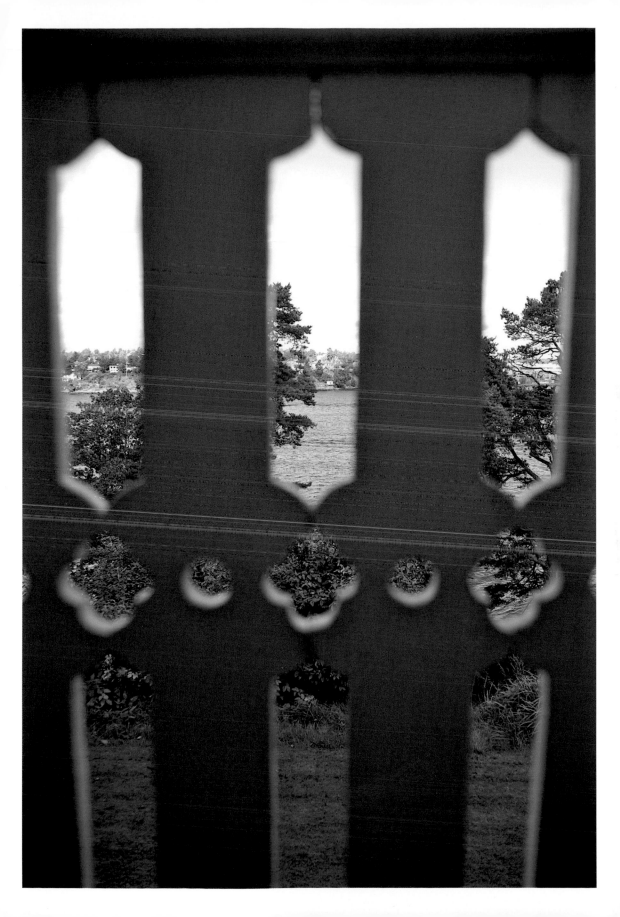

Measure Your Success

If you live and eat according to LCHQ you will see a drastic improvement. Therefore, keeping track of what happens in your body—to measure your success—is a way of motivating yourself, and to show how important it is. It also makes it more fun.

Slow-acting carbohydrates, exercise, antioxidants, and good fats will give you better insulin sensitivity, something many people need. Of the approximately 23 million Americans with diabetes, it is estimated that between 90 to 95 percent have type 2 diabetes. And there are many more who are undiagnosed, or who have pre-diabetes. Improved insulin sensitivity would lead to many people getting rid of their diabetes and people who are at risk would never develop it. Some indicators of having poor insulin sensitivity and/or diabetes are: being overweight, especially an abnormal fat repository around the waist. The classic "apple shaped" figure is an indication that a person is at risk. When you have developed diabetes, you will become abnormally hungry and thirsty and will need to go to the bathroom very frequently. You will easily become tired and will need to sleep more than usual. When the disease is far along, your vision will deteriorate and your feet and hands will often become numb.

It's easy to determine if you have poor insulin sensitivity through a standardized test at the health clinic. If you are concerned, you should definitely take the test. Walking around with high blood sugar for years causes glycation of proteins and increases the risk for deteriorated vision, cardiovascular disease, and injury to the kidneys. You could say that a high blood sugar level can speed up the aging process and your body will suffer in numerous ways.

Measure your blood pressure

Your blood pressure can best be described as the pressure your blood vessels feel when the blood circulates. A high blood pressure can cause cardiovascular disease, stroke, and brain bleeds, and a blood pressure that is too low will not provide your body with enough oxygen. If the brain doesn't receive enough oxygen, you will become dizzy and faint. The LCHQ diet and lifestyle usually optimizes your blood pressure, especially for those whose pressure is high. You often measure the systolic blood pressure when the heart contracts, which should amount to about 120 to 140 mmHg. For people with diabetes or kidney failure, it should not exceed 130 mmHg. When the heart eventually expands, the pressure diminishes, which is called diastolic pressure. It should not exceed 90 mmHg.

Blood pressure is easily measured at health clinics and even at some pharmacies.

Measure your body fat

In reality, your weight is not the most important factor when it comes to health. It's much more important to know what your body consists of. If you have a lot of muscle and little fat, you'll have a high body mass index (BMI) and would accordingly be deemed overweight. The question is whether or not star athletes would be considered fat. Of course not! They have consciously altered their body compositions to build muscle and expend superfluous fat. The result is that their well-developed muscle tissue keeps their blood sugar in check, the fat-burning process efficient, and blood fats low. Research has shown that there is a very close correlation between muscle mass and a long life/health, and this is what we should strive for—not just optimal weight.

Therefore, my advice is to measure your blood fat instead of weighing yourself to see where you currently stand, and then create a plan for the future. Men ought to have about 10 to 20 percent fat, and women should have about 20 to 30 percent. If you're outside of this range, it's time for a change.

There are many ways to measure your body fat. With a bioimpedance scale you can do it in the comfort of your home; at a gym, instructors will often use a vernier scale. A vernier scale is a form of tongs that measures how many millimeters of subcutaneous fat you have in a couple of different parts of your body. These values will then be used to calculate the total amount of body fat. However, the most reliable way of calculating body fat is a Bod Pod. Resembling an egg, you sit in this machine and the "egg" calculates how much air space your body takes up. Since a liter of fat and a liter of muscle have different weights, it can quickly calculate how much body fat you have.

The easiest and cheapest way to estimate whether or not your body composition is improving is actually through the old fashioned measuring tape. A lot of people might not lose weight when they start exercising, but the waistline, buttocks, and arms will all shrink.

If you still want to use a scale

Of course it is fine to use a scale in order to keep track of your progress, but you have to be aware of the things I just mentioned. A scale will actually only produce the most accurate number when you first reach your optimal weight and are stable. As long as the diet and exercise stay the same over a long period of time, it's a good time to weigh yourself once a week to make sure you're not slowly gaining the weight back or losing unhealthy amounts. My advice is to weigh yourself on a Sunday morning before breakfast, after a trip to the restroom. That will ensure a standardized weighing that reduces the risk of misleading results. If you weigh yourself at different times, there could be a deviation of several pounds depending on food, bathroom visits, exercise, fluids, etc.

Sleep, sweet tooth, and quality of life

Blood pressure, weight, and body fat are easy to measure, and it's easy to see how your diet affects each aspect. But LCHQ actually provides much more than that.

For example, your sleep may be affected. Has your sleep quality changed? Do you need as many hours in bed and are you actually more energetic when it's time to wake up? LCHQ is a diet that provides an adequate amount of carbohydrates to optimize your production of serotonin. This is important for a good night's sleep, since you sleep better when your body contains an adequate amount of serotonin. Even exercising works well with LCHQ and will significantly improve your sleep. Nothing reduces your stress hormones and generates good sleep as much as regular exercise.

What about hunger and cravings for sweets? Even in this regard you will see significant change. Since the LCHQ diet completely excludes refined sugar, your sweet tooth will significantly diminish. You'll surely think of sugar as something "delicious," but you'll rarely feel that irresistible craving after your sugar habit has been eliminated.

Also, don't forget to notice how your general health improves—most notably your overall energy. Most people experience their immune system working better, especially when they start taking probiotics. It's pretty easy to count the number of annual colds (which will probably be low with LCHQ). Even your overall energy will increase, since you'll have few blood sugar fluctuations and an even and constant access to that blood sugar. All in all, your overall quality of life will improve.

"In reality, your weight is not the most important factor when it comes to health. It's much more important to know what your body consists of."

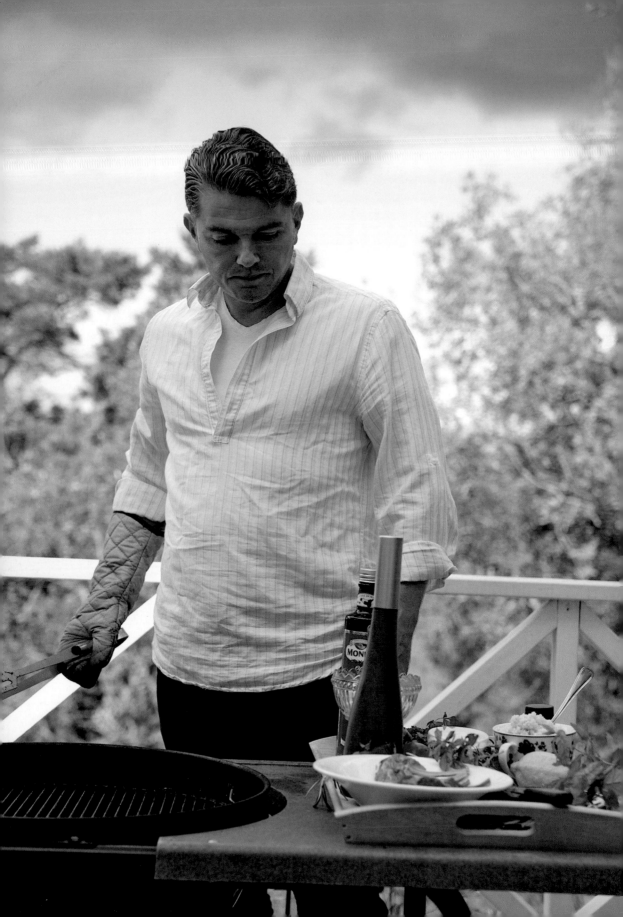

LCHQ

RECIPES

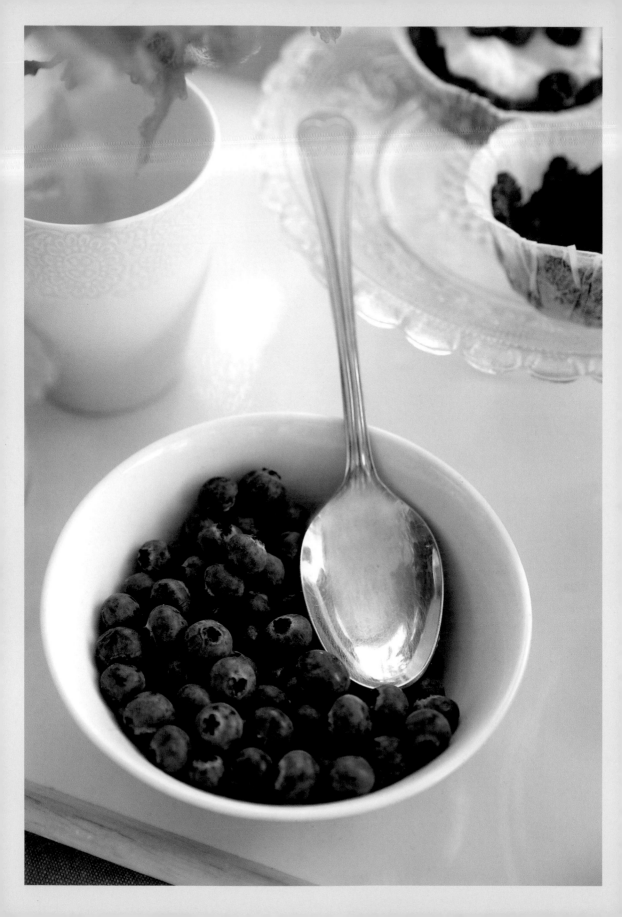

BREAKFAST

LCHQ GRANOLA

BLUEBERRY SMOOTHIE

RASPBERRY AND COCONUT SMOOTHIE

MILK-FREE SMOOTHIE

BREAKFAST OMELET

LCHQ **GRANOLA**

10 servings

3/4 cup (200 ml) pumpkin seeds
3/4 cup (200 ml) sunflower seeds
3/4 cup (200 ml) crushed flaxseed
3/4 cup (200 ml) hazelnuts
3/4 cup (200 ml) pecans
5 tsp cinnamon

Chop up all the nuts and combine all ingredients. Store in an airtight container. Serve a 1/2 cup (100 ml) of granola with 3/4 cup (200 ml) of plain yogurt along with 1/2 cup (100 ml) of raspberries.

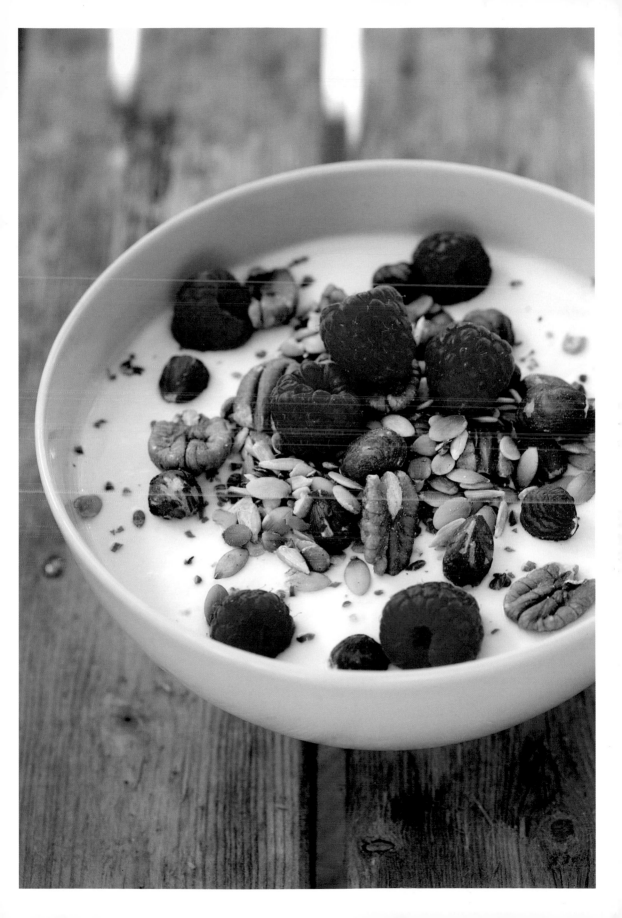

BLUEBERRY
SMOOTHIE

1 serving

**1/2 cup (125 g) plain Greek
yogurt
3/4 cup (200 ml) milk
1/2 cup (100 ml) frozen
blueberries
15 sweet almonds
1/2 tbsp peeled sesame seeds
1/2 tbsp crushed flaxseed
1 boiled egg**

Place the yogurt, milk, blueberries, almonds, and seeds in a blender and mix until it is smooth. Pour into a glass and serve with a boiled egg.

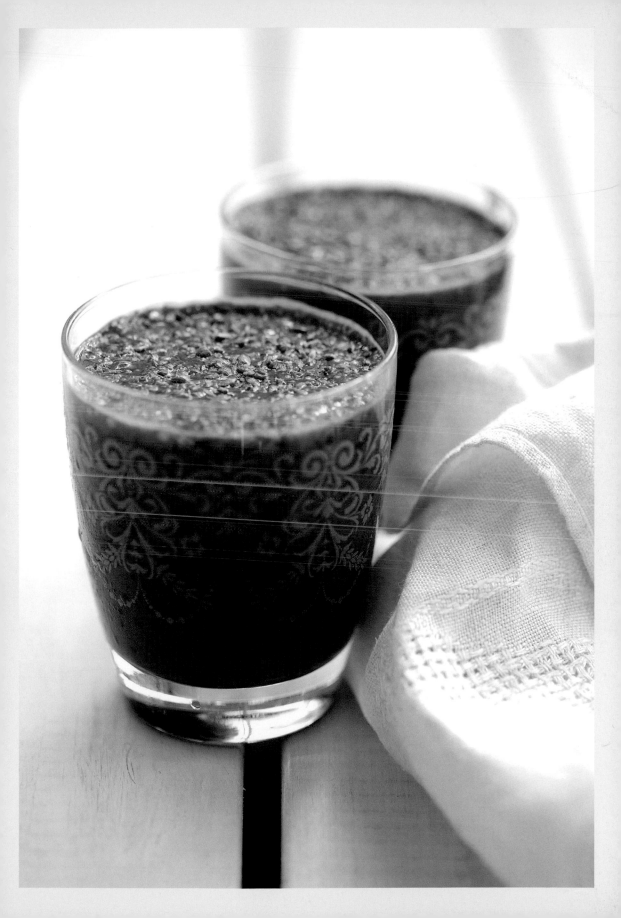

RASPBERRY AND COCONUT
SMOOTHIE

1 serving

**1/2 cup (125 g) plain
Greek yogurt
1/2 cup (100 ml) coconut milk
1/2 cup (100 ml) milk
1/2 cup (100 ml) frozen raspberries
1 tbsp pumpkin seeds**

Place all the ingredients in a blender and mix until it is smooth.

"There should be enough nutrients to feed your muscles, brain, and immune system, as well as anything else that is fighting for what is in your blood and cells."

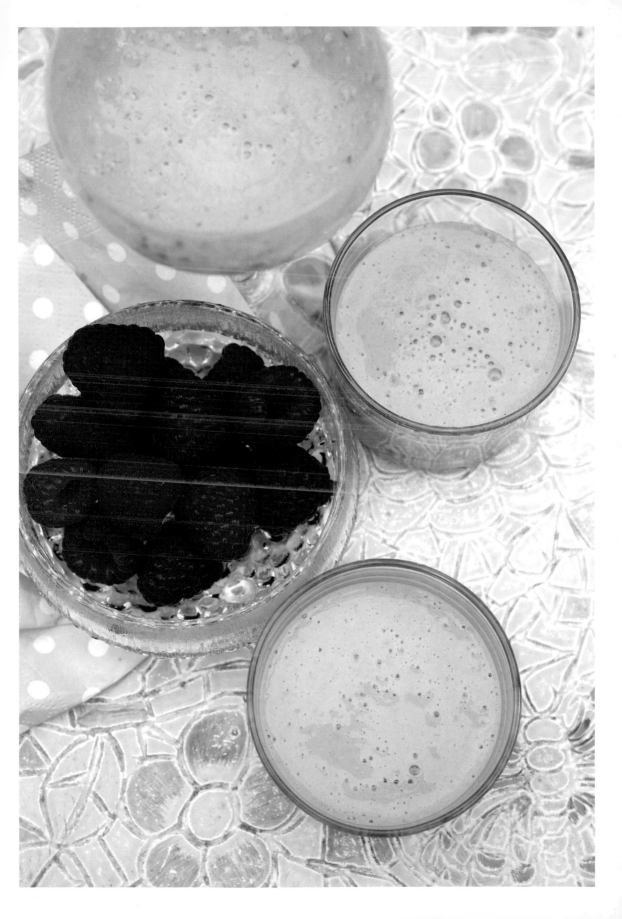

MILK-FREE **SMOOTHIE**

1 serving

3 1/2 oz (100 g) Silken tofu
1/2 cup (100 ml) coconut milk
1/2 cup (100 ml) water
1/2 cup (100 ml) frozen
blueberries
1 egg

Place all the ingredients in a blender and mix until it is smooth.

". . . coconut oil contains about 5 percent fewer calories than other sources of fat . . . Lauric acid found in coconut oil has antibacterial characteristics . . ."

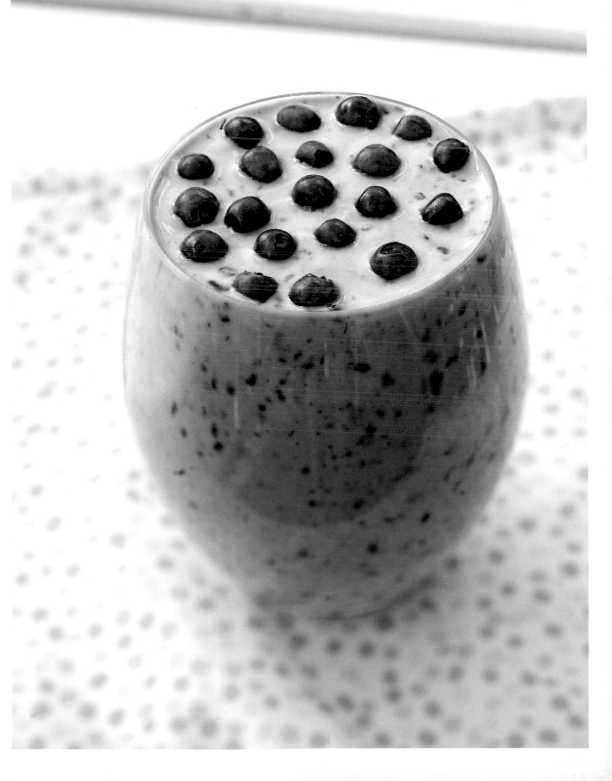

BREAKFAST OMELET

1 serving

2 eggs
2 oz (50 g) boiled ham
3 mushrooms
1 tomato
1 tbsp grated cheese
1/2 tbsp water
1 tbsp olive oil
salt and black pepper
3/4 cup (200 ml) vegetable juice

Crack the eggs in a bowl and whisk with a fork. Chop the ham and mushrooms coarsely. Core the tomato, and dice it neatly. Place the chopped ingredients in the whisked egg. Add the cheese, water, salt, and pepper. Heat the olive oil in a frying pan and pour in the egg mixture. Cook the omelet at medium heat until it has solidified. Serve with a glass of vegetable juice.

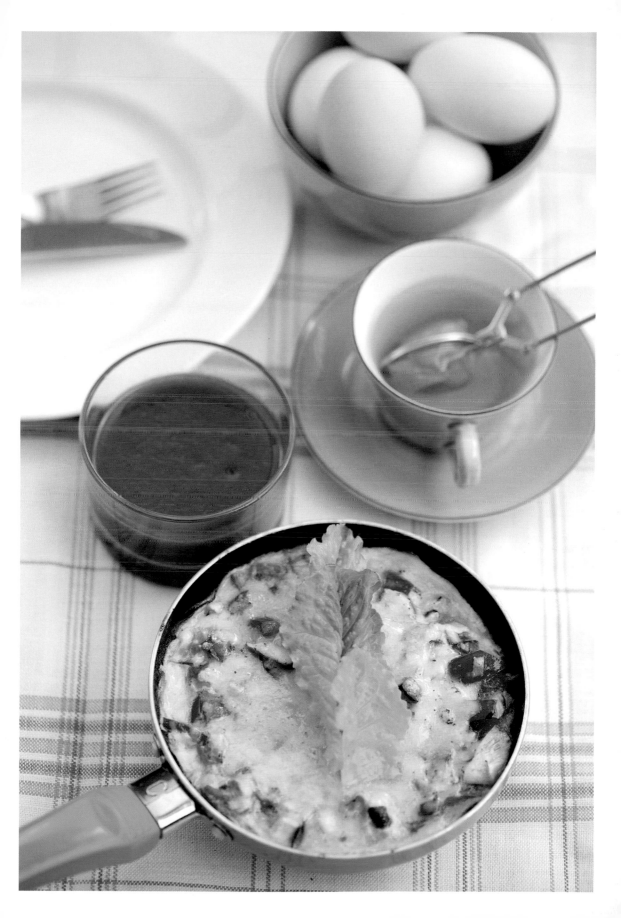

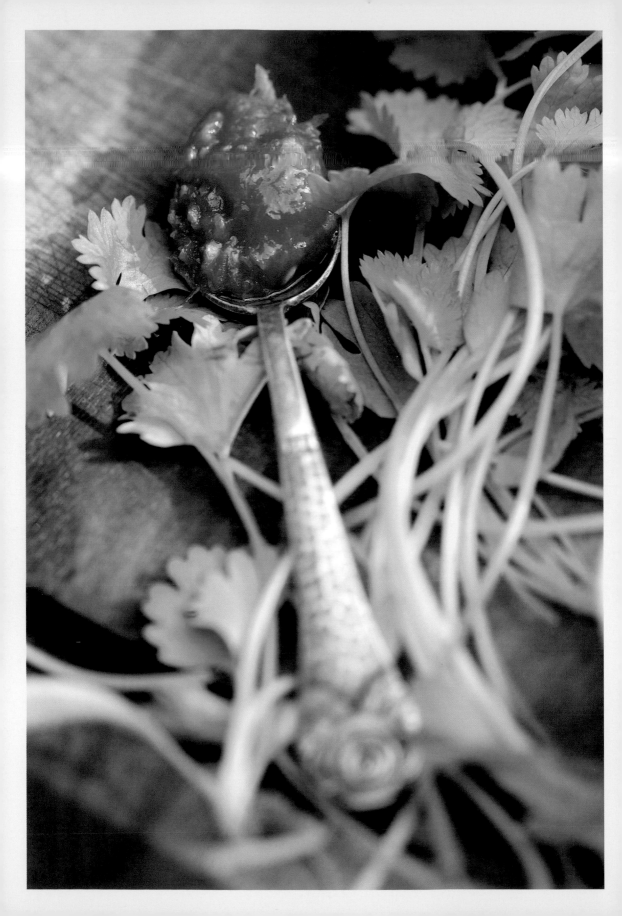

LUNCH
& DINNER

HOT CHICKEN DRUMSTICKS WITH COLESLAW

PICKLED SALMON WITH WARMED SCALLION SALAD

GRILLED SHRIMP SCAMPI WITH GREEN SALAD AND AVOCADO CREAM

GOLDEN CABBAGE PUDDING

LEMON CHICKEN WITH OVEN-BAKED VEGETABLES

FISH SOUP WITH AIOLI

LCHQ ROOT VEGETABLES WITH SALMON AND FETA

LEMONGRASS CHICKEN STIR FRY WITH A GREEN SALAD

STUFFED PEPPERS AND PORTOBELLO MUSHROOMS

MEAT-STUFFED EGGPLANTS

GRILLED RACK OF LAMB WITH TABBOULEH TOMATOES AND

   FETA CHEESE MIX

HOT **CHICKEN DRUMSTICKS**
WITH **COLESLAW**

4 servings

approx. 2 lbs (1 kg) chicken drumsticks

MARINADE
4 tbsp olive oil
3 tbsp lemon juice
1 tbsp soy sauce
1 tbsp tomato purée
2 tsp honey
1 tsp chili flakes

COLESLAW
14 oz (400 g) cabbage
2 carrots
1/4 cup pumpkin seeds

DRESSING
1/2 cup (100 ml) Greek yogurt
1 tbsp mayonnaise
1 garlic clove, pressed
1/2 tsp lemon juice
1/2 tsp mustard
1 pinch of salt
1/2 tsp black pepper

Combine all ingredients for the marinade. Marinate the drumsticks for at least an hour before cooking. Cook the drumsticks in the oven at 450°F (225°C) for approximately 30 minutes.

Finely shred the cabbage. Peel the carrots and grate them coarsely. Mix together the dressing and pour over the cabbage and carrots. Add the pumpkin seeds. Mix well. Serve with the chicken.

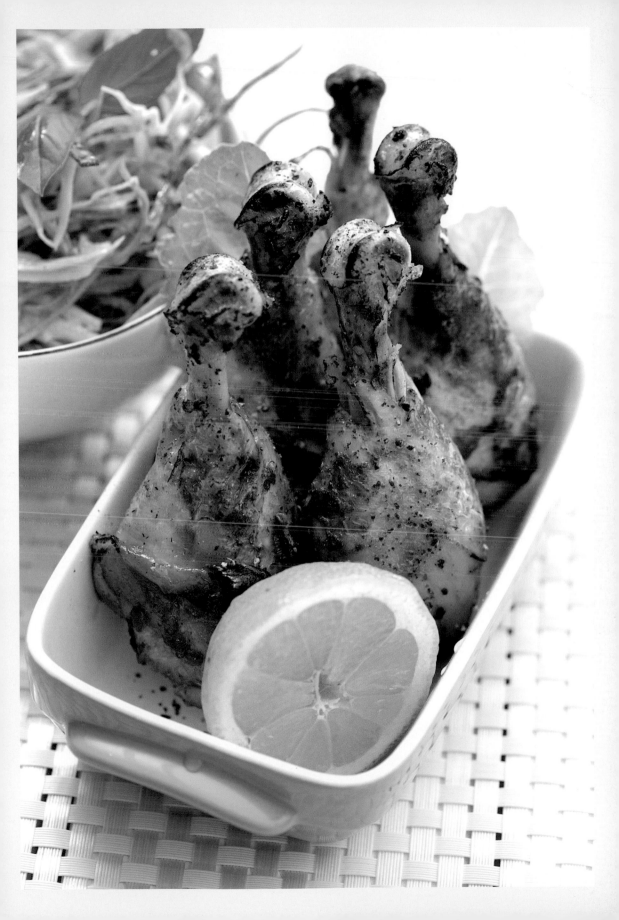

PICKLED SALMON
WITH WARMED SCALLION SALAD

4 servings

2 lbs (800 g) salmon fillets

PRESERVING JUICE
4 1/4 cups (1 liter) water
1/2 lemon (preferably organic), sliced
2 tsp salt
a few dill sprigs

DILL MAYONNAISE
3/4 cup (200 ml) crème fraiche
2 tbsp mayonnaise
3 1/2 tbsp cup (50 ml) chopped fresh dill
1 garlic clove, pressed
1/2 tsp salt

WARMED SCALLION SALAD
10 1/2 oz (300 g) romaine lettuce
1 1/2 oz (70 g) mache lettuce
17 1/2 oz (500 g) green asparagus
1 bunch of radishes
1 cup (150 g) sugar peas
2 tbsp olive oil
1 tbsp balsamic vinegar
sea salt and black pepper

Bring the preserving juice to a boil and let simmer for a couple of minutes. Cut the salmon into four equally large pieces. Remove the pot from the stove and add the fish. The preserving juice must completely cover the fish. Return the pot to the stove and let simmer while covered for about 10 minutes. Remove the fish and peel off the skin.

Mix together the dill mayonnaise.

Rinse the vegetables. Coarsely shred the lettuce. Break off the lower parts of the asparagus and cut each asparagus stalk into three pieces. Clean the radishes and slice them. Heat the olive oil in a large frying or wok. Add the asparagus, radishes, and sugar peas and stir at a high temperature without letting them change color, about 3 to 4 minutes. The vegetables should still be crispy. Add the sea salt. Place the lettuce on a large plate, top with the vegetables, balsamic vinegar, and black pepper. Mix it all together. Serve with the pickled salmon and dill mayonnaise.

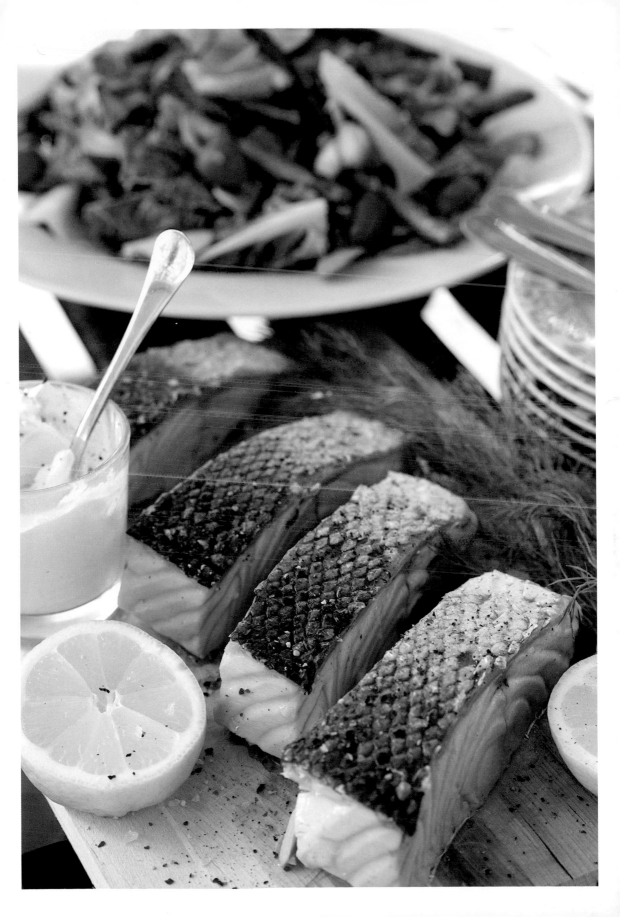

GRILLED SHRIMP SCAMPI
WITH GREEN SALAD AND AVOCADO CREAM

4 servings

1 lb (500 g) shrimp
4 skewers

MARINADE
1 red chili pepper
1/4 cup olive oil
1 lime, zest and juice
2 garlic cloves, pressed
1 tsp grated ginger
a pinch of salt

AVOCADO CREAM
4 avocados
1/4 cup Greek yogurt
2 tsp lime juice
2 garlic cloves, pressed
salt and black pepper

GREEN SALAD
10 1/2 oz (300 g) romaine lettuce
3 1/2 oz (100 g) green leaves
20 cherry tomatoes
1 red onion
10 1/2 oz (300 g) marinated artichokes
2 tbsp olive oil
1 tbsp vinegar

Soak the skewers in cold water. Split the chili pepper vertically, remove the core and walls, and finely chop what is left. Mix the marinade and marinate the shrimp for an hour. Pierce the shrimp with the skewers.

Mash the avocado and mix in the yogurt, lime, and garlic. Add salt and pepper to taste.

Split the tomatoes. Cut the onion into thin slices. Distribute the lettuce on four plates, and top with slices of onion, tomatoes, and artichokes. Drizzle the olive oil and vinegar on top. Distribute the avocado cream into four small cups and place them on the plates.

Grill the shrimp on a grill or in the oven. If using an oven, set the oven to broil and place the skewers close to the top for about 5 minutes. Turn them over once during the grilling.

Place the skewers on the plates with the salad and serve.

Tip: If you can't find raw shrimp in the store, buy frozen. Just heat it up quickly in a frying pan or in the oven after marinating.

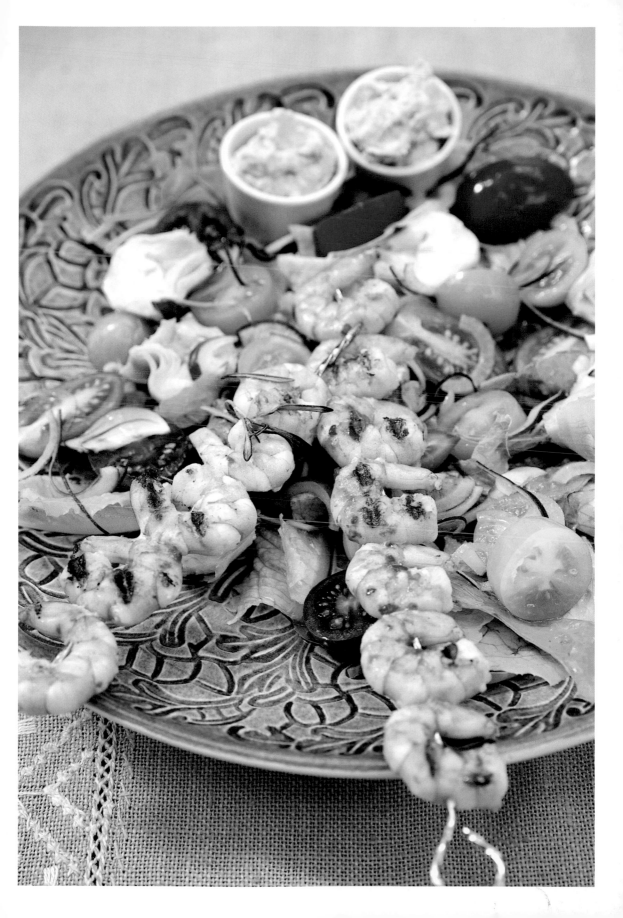

GOLDEN **CABBAGE PUDDING**

4 servings

21 oz (600 g) cabbage
1 lb (500 g) ground venison
(or ground beef)
1 onion
2 tbsp olive oil
1 cube of beef bouillon
1 tsp salt
black and white pepper
1/2 cup (100 ml) cream
1/4 cup (50 ml) uncooked whole grain rice
3/4 cup (200 ml) frozen cranberries

Finely shred the cabbage and boil it in a saucepan with 3/4 cup (200 ml) water until the cabbage is soft (approximately 15 minutes). While the cabbage is boiling, in a frying pan, sear the ground venison or beef and onion with the oil. Add bouillon, salt, and pepper to taste. Pour the meat into the saucepan with the cabbage and add the cream and rice. Mix well.

Place the mixture in a baking pan and put in the center of the oven at 400°F (200°C). Let it cook for approximately 40 minutes; stir occasionally. Serve with frozen cranberries; if the frozen cranberries are too sour for your taste, sweeten with a bit of honey.

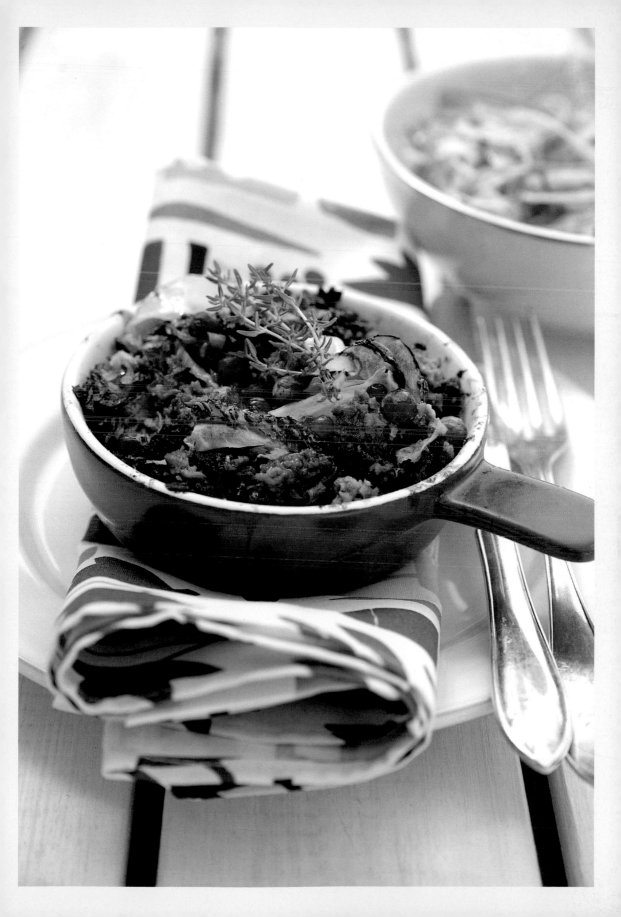

LEMON CHICKEN
WITH OVEN-BAKED VEGETABLES

4 servings

approx. 2 2/3 lbs (1.2 kg) diced chicken thighs (with skin and bone)

MARINADE
1 lemon (preferably organic), zest and juice
1/4 cup olive oil
1 tbsp soy sauce
a pinch of turmeric
a pinch of black pepper

OVEN-BAKED VEGETABLES
4 small fennel stalks
8 parsnips
1 large red onion
12 mushrooms
8 garlic cloves
20 green olives
16 cherry tomatoes
salt and pepper

FETA CHEESE MIX
2/3 cup (150 g) feta cheese
1/2 cup (100 ml) Greek yogurt
1 tsp olive oil
black pepper

Mix the marinade for the chicken and let it marinate for at least 30 minutes to an hour. Clean the fennel and split each stalk into 4 parts. Peel and cut each parsnip into 4 parts, peel and cut the onion, divide up the mushrooms, and peel the garlic cloves.

In a baking pan, combine the vegetables (except for the tomatoes, mushrooms, and olives) with the chicken and the marinade. Stir thoroughly with your hands and bake in the oven at 450°F (225°C). After 20 minutes, add the tomatoes, mushrooms, and olives and continue to cook until the chicken is done, which should take about 10 minutes. Add salt and pepper to taste.

Mash the feta cheese with a fork. Pour in the yogurt and olive oil and stir. Add salt and pepper to taste. Serve the feta cheese mix with the chicken and vegetables.

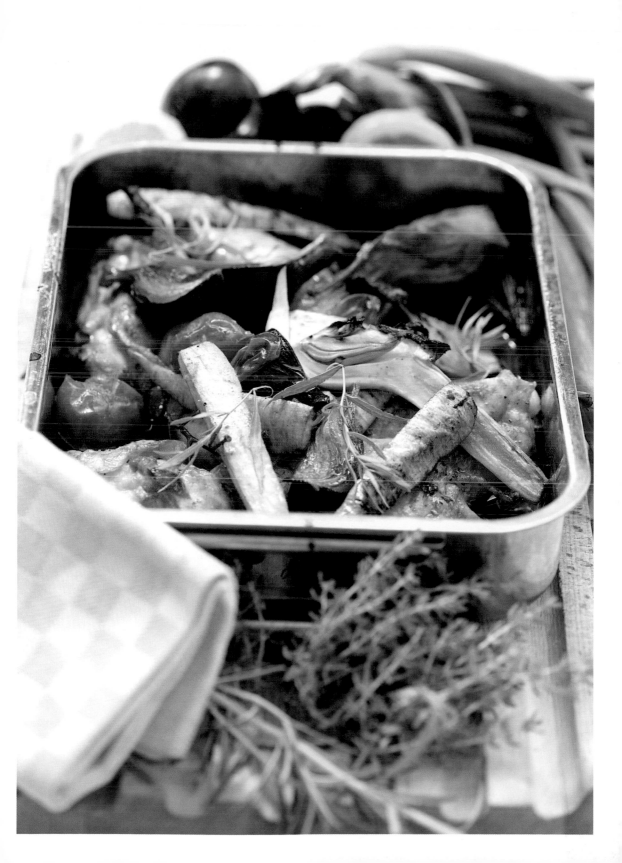

FISH SOUP WITH AIOLI

4 servings

2/3 lb (300 g) salmon fillet
2/3 lb (300 g) white fish fillet (e.g. cod or
pollock)
1/3 lb (150 g) peeled shrimp
2 tbsp olive oil
3 garlic cloves
1/2 leek
1 fennel stalk
2 carrots
2 parsnips
1 pinch, (1/2 a packet) of saffron
1 can of canned cherry tomatoes
4 1/4 cup (1 liter) water
3 tbsp fish stock
2 tbsp tomato purée
1 tsp dried thyme
a pinch of black pepper
salt

AIOLI
1/4 cup crème fraîche
1/4 cup mayonnaise
2 garlic cloves, pressed
salt

Heat the olive oil in a large saucepan. Finely chop the garlic and fry in the oil—but be careful not to sear it. Add in the thinly sliced leek, coarsely chopped fennel, and thinly sliced carrots and parsnips. Fry until the vegetables have softened slightly and are shiny. Add the saffron and fry for a short while. Add the cherry tomatoes, water, fish stock, tomato puree, thyme, and black pepper. Let the mixture boil until the vegetables are soft.

Add the fish and let simmer for a couple of minutes. Add the shrimp, remove from the stove, and add salt to taste. Stir together the ingredients for the aioli and add salt to taste.

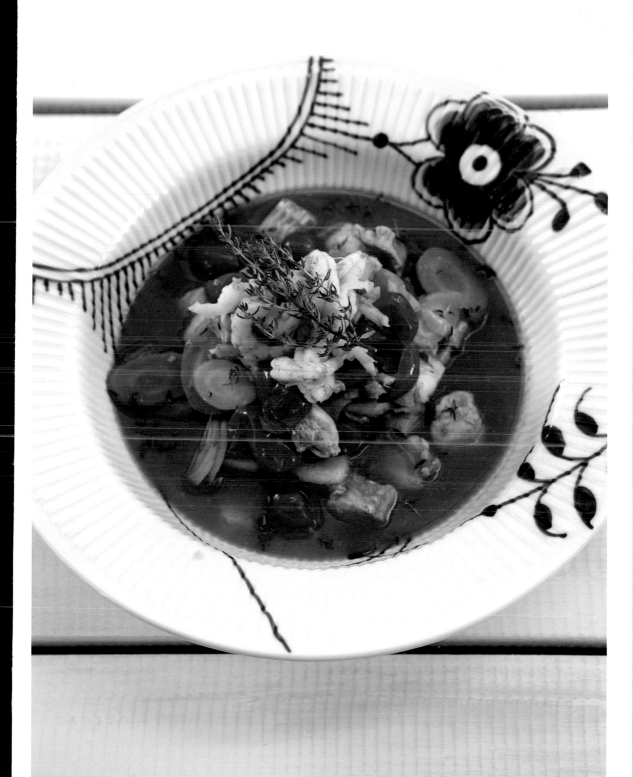

LCHQ ROOT VEGETABLES
WITH **SALMON AND FETA**

4 servings

1 1/3 lbs (600 g) salmon fillet
2/3 lb (300 g) beets
2/3 lb (300 g) parsley root
2/3 lb (300 g) celery root
2/3 lb (300 g) turnips (alt. kohlrabi)
4 tbsp olive oil
1 tsp dried herbs, e.g. Herbes de Provence
salt and black pepper
2/3 cup (150 g) feta cheese

Peel the root vegetables and cut them into equally large chunks. Place them in a baking pan and drizzle with olive oil. Sprinkle the herbs on top and add salt and pepper to taste. Stir so that the spices and oil are thoroughly mixed. Bake in the oven at 450°F (225°C) for about 25 minutes. Reduce the heat to 400°F (200°C) and place a baking sheet with the fish in the oven. Continue baking the vegetables and the fish for 15–20 minutes.

Sprinkle the feta cheese over the root vegetables and season the fish with salt.

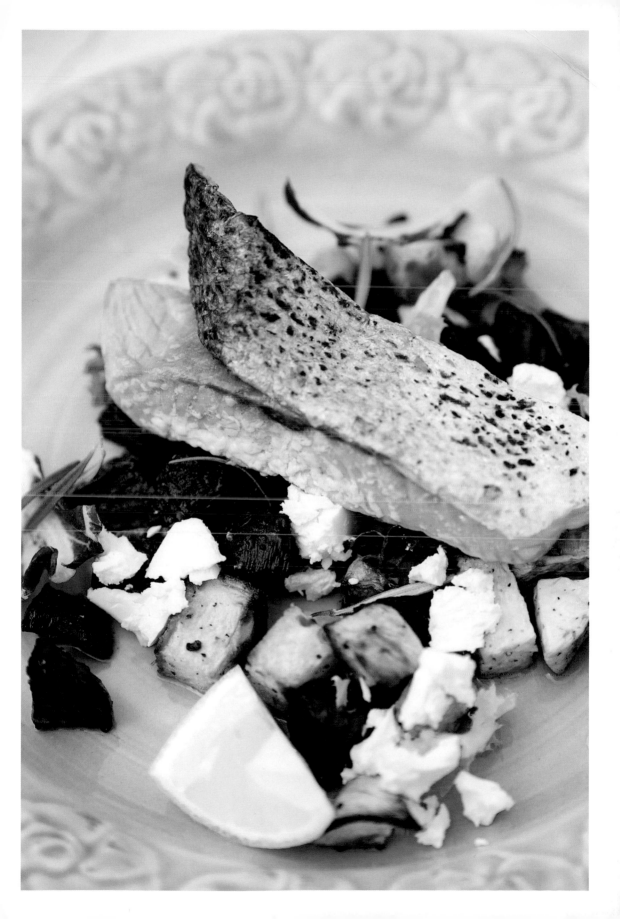

LEMONGRASS
CHICKEN STIR FRY
WITH **A GREEN SALAD**

4 servings

1 1/3 lbs (600 g) chicken thigh fillets
3/4 cup (80 g) roasted cashews

MARINADE

1 red chili pepper
1 lemongrass stalk
4 garlic cloves
4 tbsp canola oil
4 tbsp Thai fish sauce

SALAD

1 squash (alt. 1 cucumber)
2 peppers of different colors
3 1/2 oz (100 g) baby spinach

DRESSING

2 tbsp canola oil
1 tbsp squeezed lime
herb salt

Split the chili, scrape out the seeds, and finely shred it. Lightly pound the white part of the lemongrass stalk and finely chop it. Peel and finely chop the garlic. Mix the marinade.

Cut the chicken into small slices and let them marinate for half an hour. Fry the chicken in a wok or large frying pan with the marinade until it is fully cooked, for approximately 5 minutes. Add the nuts.

Cut the peppers and the squash into chunks and mix with the spinach. Prepare the dressing and pour on top.

Tips: If you want a warm salad, you can quickly heat the salad in the wok, but be carefully that the vegetables maintain their crispiness.

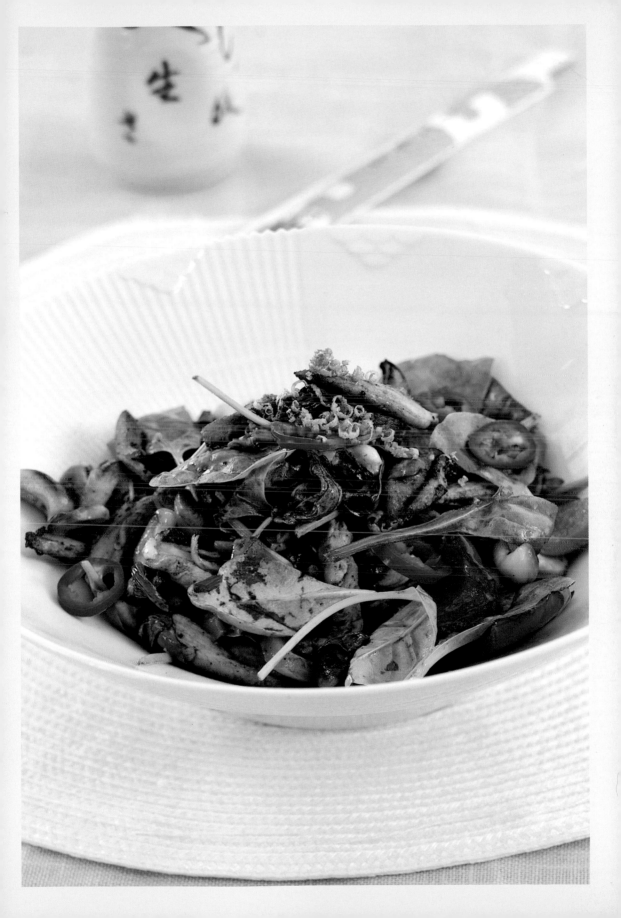

STUFFED **PEPPERS** AND
PORTOBELLO MUSHROOMS

4 servings

4 red bell peppers
4 portobello mushrooms
1lb (500 g) ground beef (10% fat)
1 red onion
2 garlic cloves
2 tbsp olive oil
2 tbsp tomato purée
2 tsp pizza seasoning
2 pinches of salt
a pinch of black pepper
a pinch of white pepper
approx. 5 drops of tabasco sauce
1 tbsp olive oil for brushing
1 1/3 cups (300 ml) grated cheese

Chop the onion and garlic and fry quickly in oil. Add the beef and sear it. Add the spices. Cut off the tops of the peppers and remove the core and seeds. Wash off the mushrooms and cut off the stems. Brush the mushrooms with olive oil. Distribute the beef into the peppers and into the mushroom caps and sprinkle the grated cheese on top. Bake in the oven at 450°F (225°C) for 15 to 20 minutes.

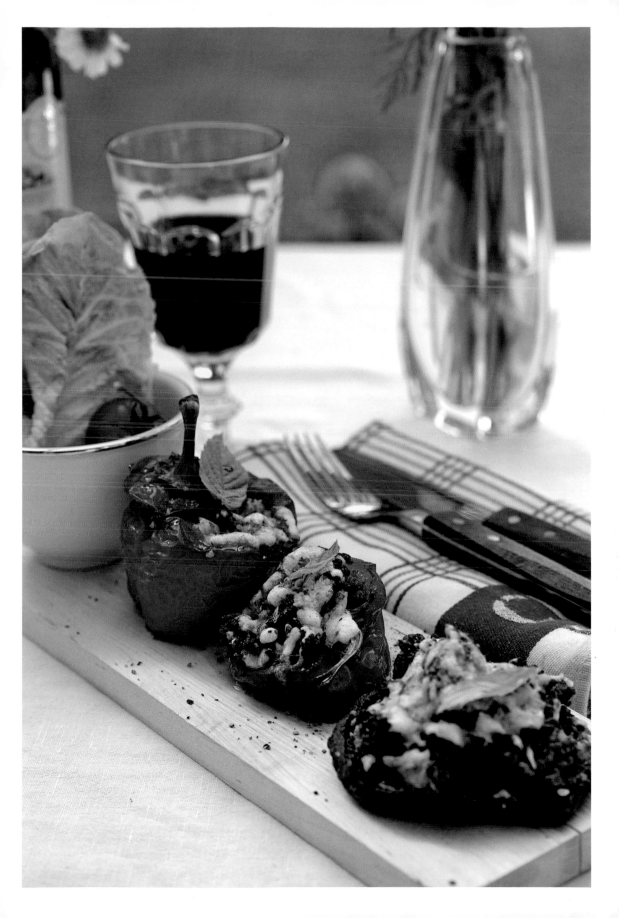

MEAT-STUFFED
EGGPLANTS

4 servings

4 eggplants
1lb (500 g) ground beef (max. 10% fat)
1 large onion
4 tbsp olive oil
1 tsp curry
2 pinches of salt
1 1/3 cups (300 ml) grated cheese

Halve the eggplants lengthwise and carefully scoop out the flesh. Dice the eggplant flesh. Peel and chop the onion. Heat the olive oil in a frying pan and fry the onion and eggplant flesh for about 5 minutes, until they are soft. Remove from the pan and sear the meat. Season with curry and salt to taste. Combine the meat and the vegetables, and place in the eggplant halves. Sprinkle grated cheese on top and bake in the oven at 400°F (200°C) for about 30 minutes, until the eggplant flesh is soft.

Ideally, serve the stuffed eggplants topped with lettuce, cucumber, and tomatoes.

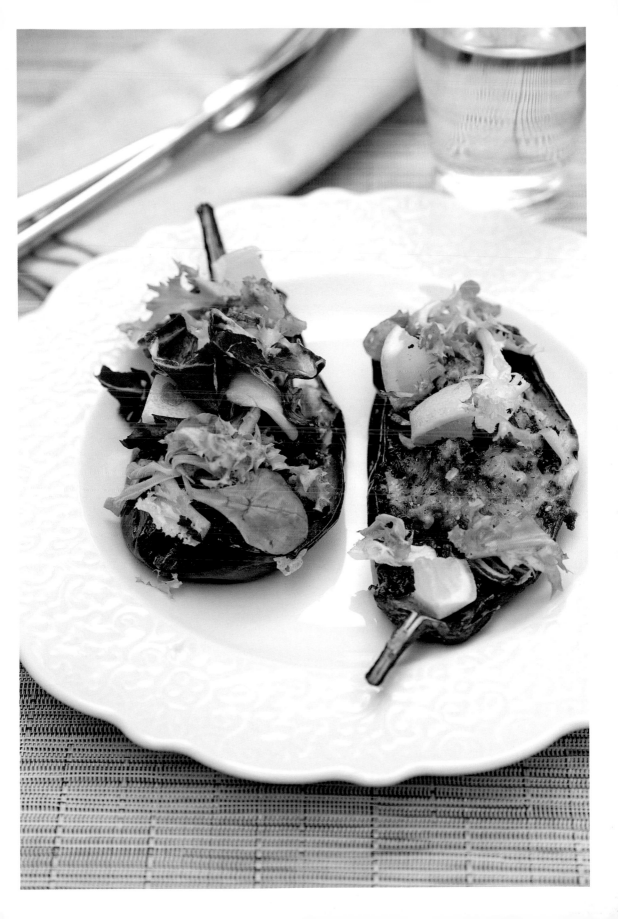

GRILLED **RACK OF LAMB**
WITH **TABBOULEH TOMATOES**
AND **FETA CHEESE MIX**

4 servings

2 1/4 lbs (1 kg) racks of lamb

MARINADE
2/3 cup (150 ml) olive oil
8 garlic cloves, pressed
1 tbsp Herbes de Provence
1 pinch of salt

TABBOULEH TOMATOES
4 large tomatoes
1/2 cup (100 ml) bulgur
1 red onion
2 tbsp fresh parsley, chopped
1 tbsp fresh mint, chopped
2 tbsp freshly squeezed lemon juice
salt and black pepper

FETA CHEESE MIX
2/3 cup (150 g) feta cheese
1/2 cup (100 ml) Greek yogurt
1 tsp olive oil
black pepper

Prepare the marinade and marinate the split lamb racks for at least a couple of hours. Remove the excess marinade before grilling to prevent the oil from dripping down onto the flame. Grill.

Soak the bulgur in water for half an hour. Halve the tomatoes and remove the cores. Peel and finely chop the onions. Remove any excess water not absorbed by the bulgur. You can squeeze out that last bit with your hands. Mix the bulgur with the herbs, onion, oil, and lemon juice. Add salt and pepper to taste. Stuff the tomato halves with the bulgur mixture and place them in a baking dish. Top each tomato with a couple of drops of oil. Bake in the oven at 450°F (225°C) for 15 to 20 minutes, until the tomatoes have gained some color. You can cover the dish with aluminum foil to keep the surface of the food from burning.

Mash the feta cheese with a fork. Pour in the yogurt and olive oil and mix until smooth. Season with black pepper to taste.

Serve the racks of lamb with the tomatoes and feta cheese mix. Serve with a green salad.

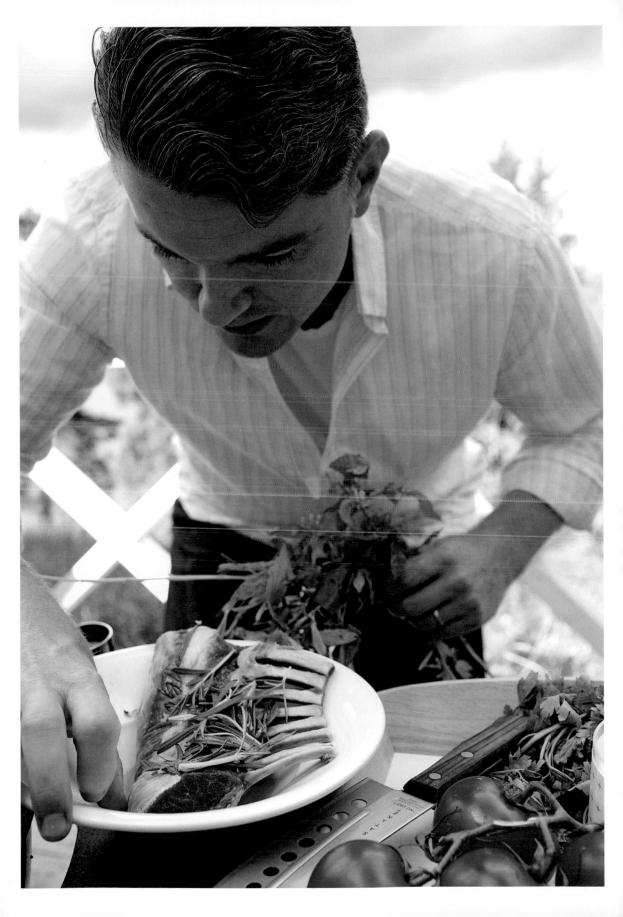

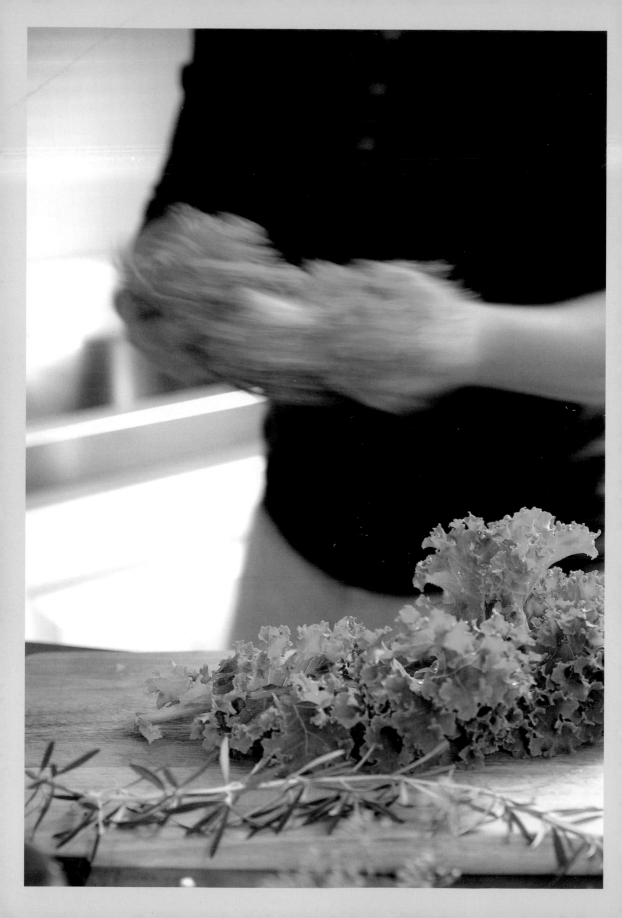

QUICK MEALS

HOT TUNA OMELET

TOFU STIR FRY

SUMMER SALAD WITH MACKEREL, EGG, AND PEAS

LCHQ MIX

HOT **TUNA OMELET**

1 serving

3 eggs
2.6 oz (75 g) canned tuna in water
1/2 onion
1/2 red chili pepper
10 leaves of fresh basil
4 green olives
1 tbsp water
a pinch of salt
a pinch of black pepper
1 tbsp olive oil
7 cherry tomatoes
2 tbsp grated cheese

Remove the tuna from the can and break it into small pieces with a fork. Chop the onion, halve and scrape the seeds from the chili pepper, and slice it thinly. Shred the basil and olives. Slice the tomatoes.

Crack the eggs into a bowl and add the tuna, chili pepper, basil, olives, water, salt, and black pepper. Lightly whisk with a fork. Heat the olive oil in a frying pan, add the onion, and fry for a short while without letting the onion brown. Pour in the egg mixture and reduce to medium heat. Let the egg solidify slightly. Add the tomatoes and cheese, and cook until the omelet is completely solidified. Make sure it doesn't burn (shake the pan occasionally to prevent this).

Serve with a handful of green leaves, such as baby spinach or arugula.

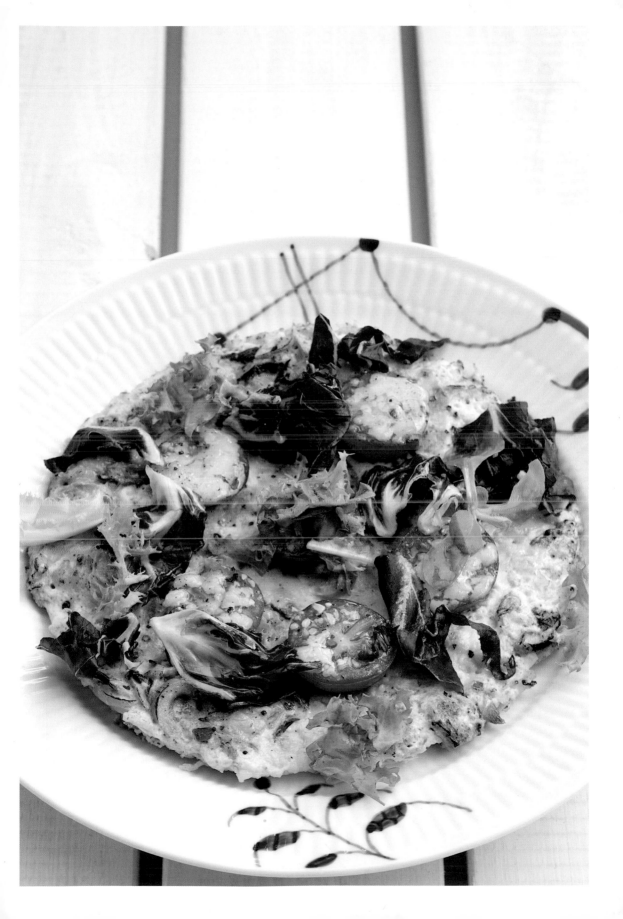

TOFU STIR FRY

1 serving

4 1/2 oz (125 g) tofu
1/2 red chili pepper
2 tbsp canola oil
1 garlic clove, pressed
1/2 tsp grated ginger
1 carrot
1/2 cup (100 ml) frozen broccoli
2 1/2 oz (70 g) green beans
2 1/2 oz (70 g) shiitake mushrooms
2 tsp soy sauce
a couple of drops of sesame oil

Dice the tofu. Split the chili pepper and scrape out the seeds. If you want it spicy, leave the seeds in. Heat 1 tablespoon of canola oil in a wok or large frying pan. Add the garlic, ginger, and tofu, and fry for about 3 minutes.

Remove the tofu. Pour 1 tablespoon of canola oil into the frying pan and add the thinly sliced carrot sticks, broccoli, green beans, mushrooms, and chili pepper. Fry for another 3 minutes. Place the tofu in the wok one more time and add 1 to 2 teaspoons of soy sauce and a couple drops of sesame oil.

Tip: You can substitute the fresh chili with chili paste (sambal oelek, for example), and the shiitake mushrooms with wild edible mushrooms, if you desire.

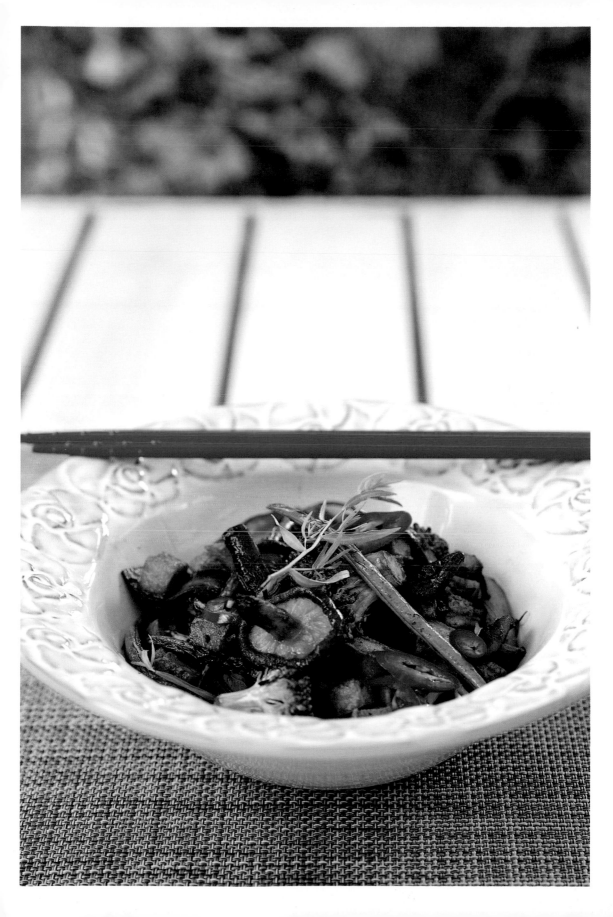

SUMMER SALAD

WITH MACKEREL, EGG, AND PEAS

1 serving

**1/4 lb (120 g) smoked pepper
mackerel fillet
3 1/2 oz (100 g) romaine lettuce
2 tbsp Greek yogurt
5 small vine tomatoes
1 softboiled egg
10 sugar snap peas**

Rinse and coarsely shred the lettuce. Arrange it on the plate. Chop the mackerel finely and stir it into the yogurt. Wedge the tomatoes and the egg. Arrange them on the plate. Remove the peas from the pod. If you cannot find fresh peas, frozen will work just as well.

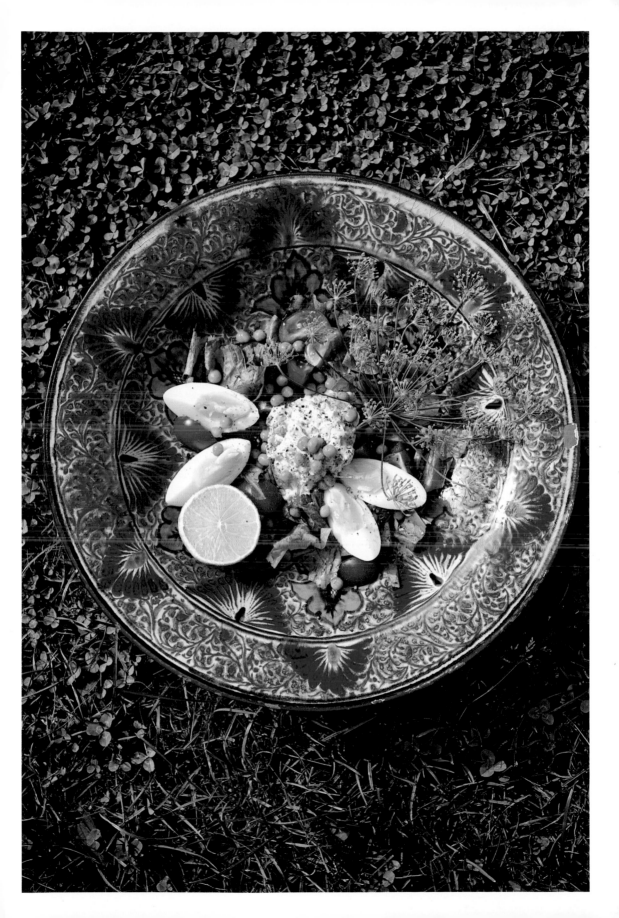

LCHQ **MIX**

2 servings

1/2 lb (240 g) frozen, shredded
venison
3/4 lb (400 g) kohlrabi
1 red bell pepper
1 onion
1 1/4 oz (35 g) coconut oil
2 eggs
salt and pepper

Peel and dice the kohlrabi. Core and dice the bell pepper. Chop the onion. Heat approximately 1 tsp of the coconut oil in a nonstick frying pan. Add the frozen venison. As it cooks, be sure to break up the meat with a wooden fork so that it sears evenly. Remove the meat from the pan and chop it finely.

Add the vegetables to the frying pan and pour in most of the coconut oil (save about 1 teaspoon) and fry at high heat for approximately 1 minute so that the surfaces are cooked. Reduce the heat to medium and fry for about 10 minutes, stirring as needed. Return the meat to the pan to heat beside the vegetables. Season with salt and pepper to taste. Distribute the mixture onto two plates. Heat the rest of the coconut oil and fry the eggs sunny side up. Top each plate with an egg.

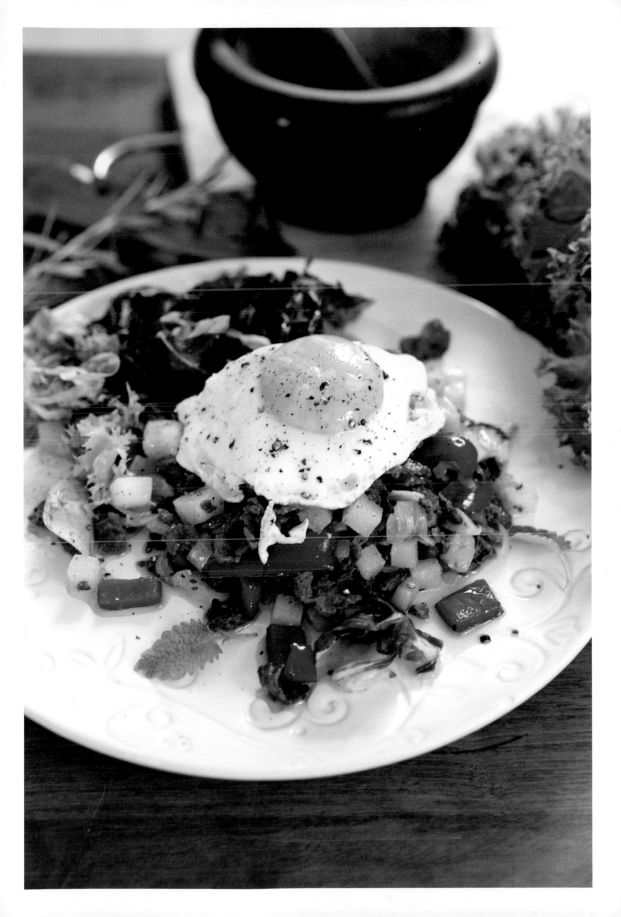

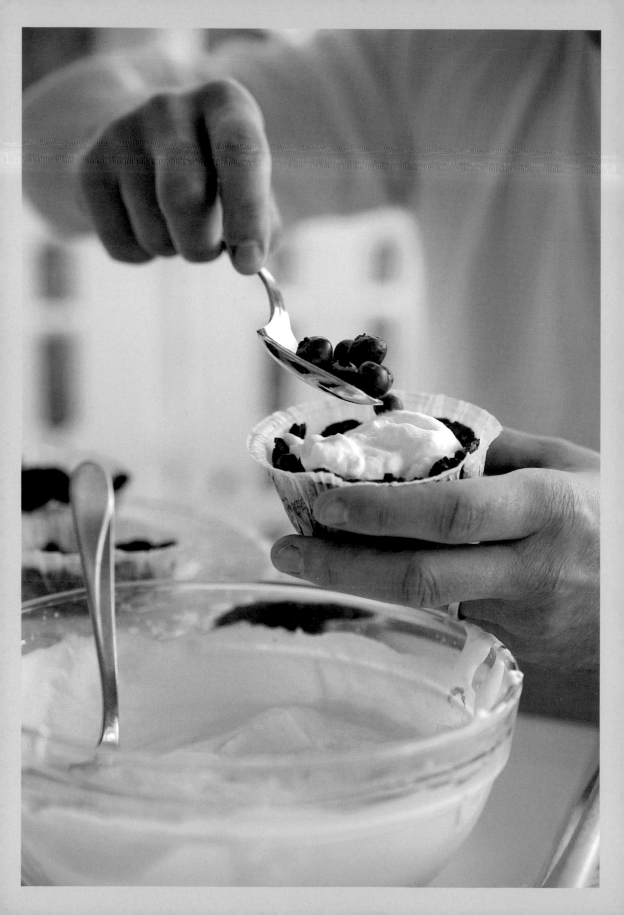

SWEETS
& DESSERTS

BLUEBERRY BEADS

GOJI BEADS

STRAWBERRY ICE CREAM WITH

  CHOCOLATE FLAKES

SIMPLE CHEESECAKE

BLUEBERRY PIE

BLUEBERRY
BEADS

approx. 15

3 1/2 tbsp (50 ml) sweet almonds
2 tbsp dried, plain blueberries
2 tbsp pumpkin seeds
2 tbsp water
3/4 oz (20 g) dark chocolate
(min. 70% cacao)
2 tbsp coconut flakes

Combine the almonds, blueberries, pumpkin seeds, and water in a food processor and mix until it becomes a smooth paste. Roll into little beads.

Melt the chocolate over a pot of boiling water and let it cool for a couple of minutes before rolling the beads in the chocolate. Roll half of the chocolate beads in the coconut flakes. Place the beads on a baking sheet and refrigerate so they solidify. The beads will keep in the refrigerator for a couple of days.

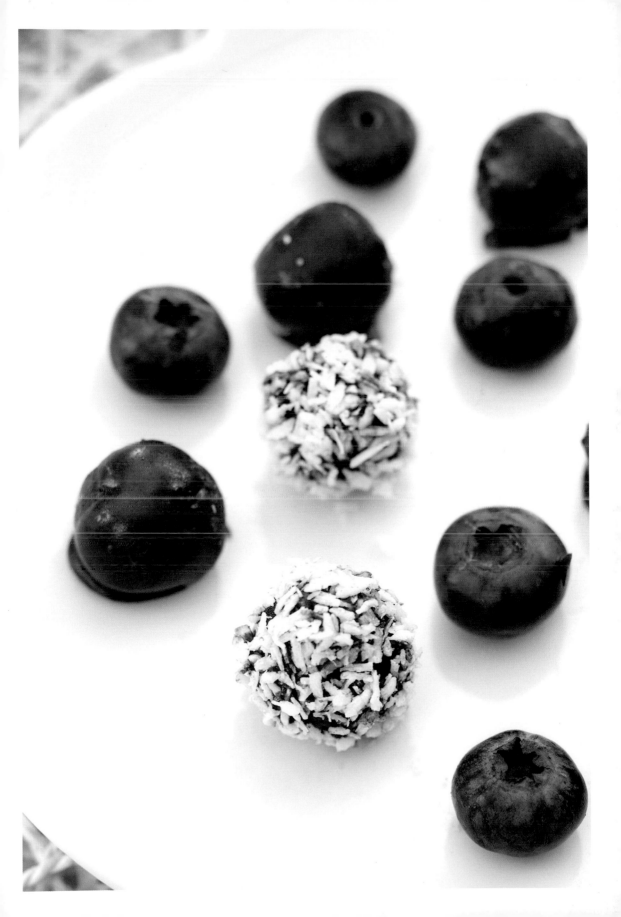

GOJI BEADS

approx. 15

3 1/2 tbsp (50 ml) sweet almonds
2 tbsp dried goji berries
2 tbsp pumpkin seeds
2 tbsp berry juice
3/4 oz (20 g) dark chocolate (85% cacao)
1–2 tsp chili flakes, optional

Soak the goji berries in the berry juice for half an hour until the liquid is absorbed. Then, place the almonds, goji berries, and pumpkin seeds in a food processor and mix until it becomes a smooth paste. Roll into beads.

Melt the chocolate over a pot of boiling water and let it cool for a couple of minutes before rolling the beads. If you like spicy desserts, you can sprinkle a couple of chili flakes on top of each bead. Place the beads on a baking sheet and refrigerate until they solidify. The beads will keep in the refrigerator for a couple of days.

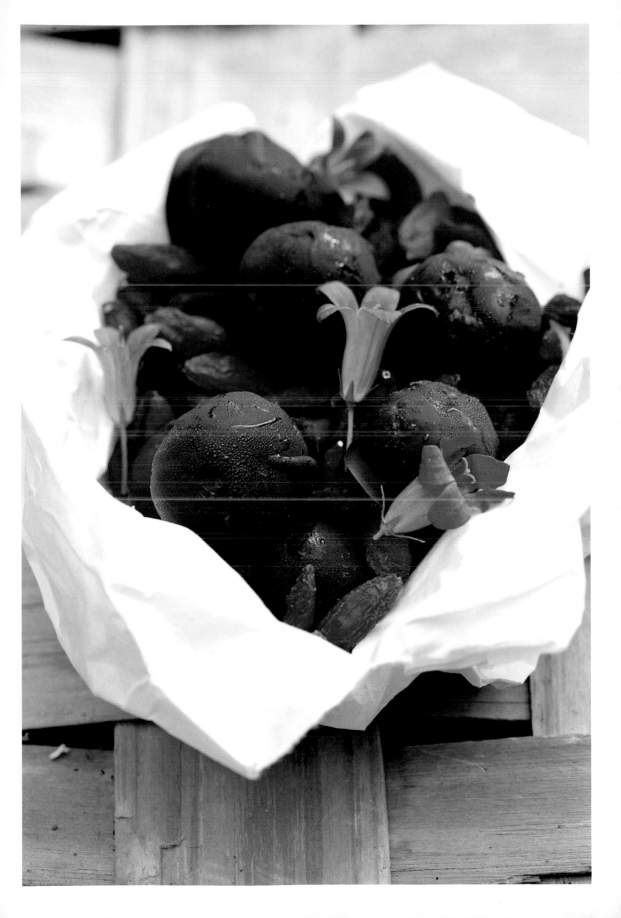

STRAWBERRY ICE CREAM
WITH CHOCOLATE FLAKES

1 serving

2 cups (125 g) Greek yogurt
2/3 cup (150 ml) frozen strawberries
1/2 oz (10 g) dark chocolate (85% cacao)

Place the yogurt and strawberries in a blender and blend until it smooth. Finely chop the chocolate and pour it over the mixture. Pour the strawberry mix into a freezer-safe container and chill in the freezer for about an hour. This will give it the perfect texture and it can be consumed immediately afterward!

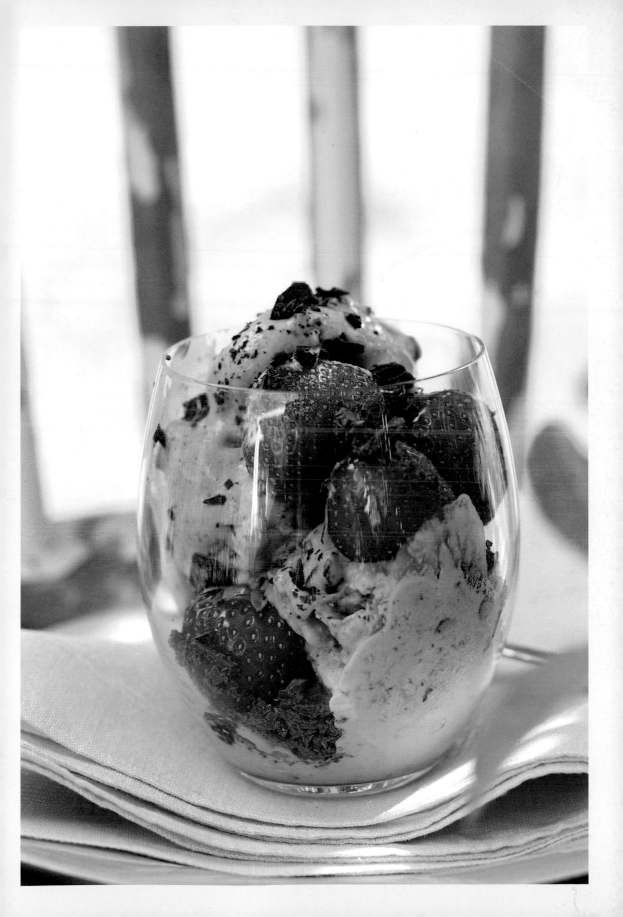

SIMPLE
CHEESECAKE

4 cups (250 g) cottage cheese
15 sweet almonds
2 eggs
1/2 cup (100 ml) cream
1 3/4 cups (400 ml) frozen raspberries
1/2 cup (100 ml) whipped cream

Drain the cottage cheese. Finely chop the almonds. In a bowl, whisk the eggs with a fork. Mix the cottage cheese, cream, and almonds. Pour the batter into a buttered baking dish. Bake in the oven at 350°F (175°C) for about 35 minutes, or until the cake has a golden brown color. If you're using a number of small ramekins instead of one large dish, the cooking time will be somewhat shorter.

Serve with raspberries and a dollop of whipped cream.

Tips: Add a pinch of saffron to the batter to make the cheesecake into a traditional Swedish "Gotland" saffron pancake. Serve with whipped cream and fresh berries. Or sprinkle cinnamon on top so the finished cake tastes like rice pudding. You can also add seeds from half a vanilla pod to the batter before baking it.

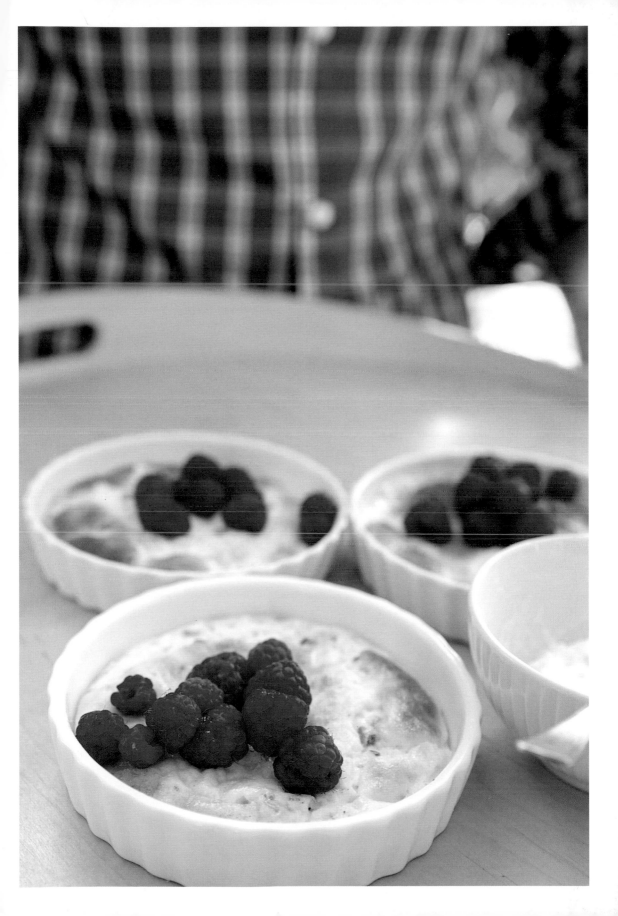

BLUEBERRY PIE

1/2 cup (100 ml) hazelnuts
1/2 cup (100 ml) pecans
1 egg
1/2 tbsp psyllium husk
2 tbsp water
1 tsp liquid honey
1 tsp coconut oil
1/2 cup (100 ml) whipped cream
3/4 cup (200 ml) fresh blueberries

Grind the nuts in a food processor until they reaches a flour-like consistency. Add the egg, psyllium husk, water, and honey. Let the mixture rest for approximately 10 minutes. Grease four individual molds with coconut oil and distribute the batter evenly. Bake in the oven at 400°F (200°C) for approximately 20 minutes. Let the pies cool. Whip the cream and dollop on top of the pies. Garnish with blueberries.

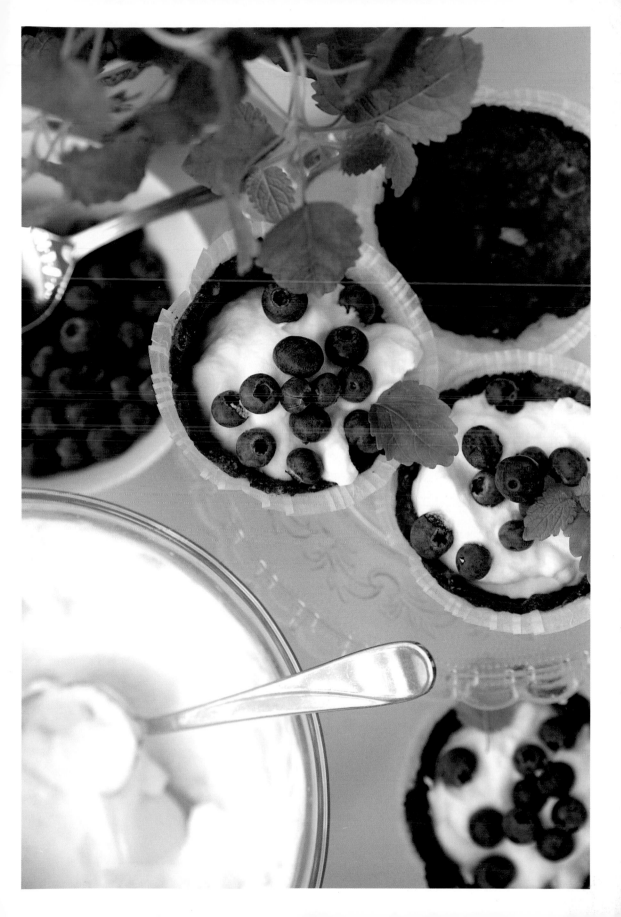

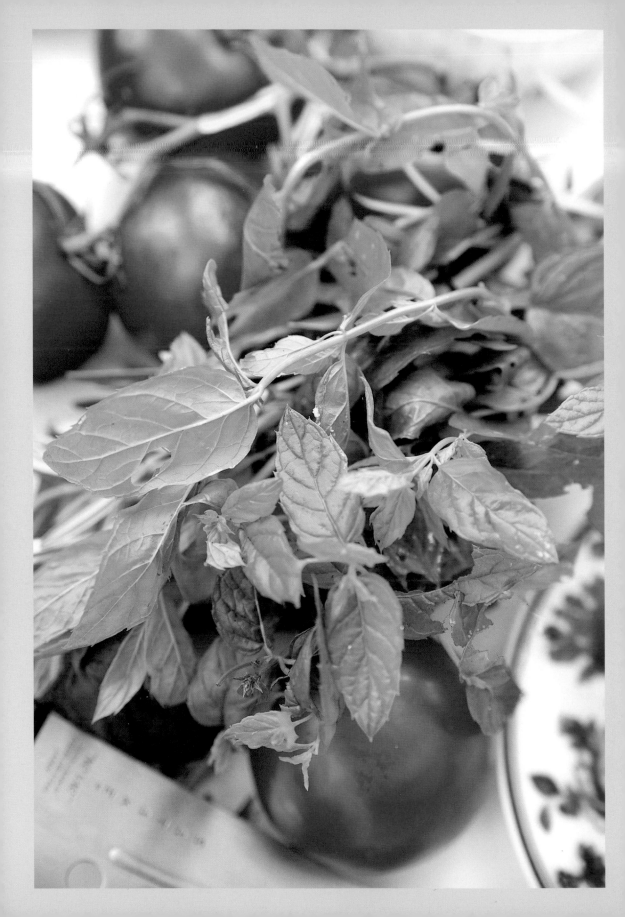

SNACKS

3
AVOCADO SNACKS

1/2 avocado
1 1/2 oz (40 g) cocktail shrimp
1 tbsp fresh dill
1/2 tbsp mayonnaise
1/2 tbsp crème fraîche

Coarsely chop the shrimp. Mix all of the ingredients and fill up the avocado skin.

1/2 avocado
1 oz (25 g) cocktail shrimp
1/2 tomato
1/2 tbsp chopped fresh cilantro
1/2 tbsp mayonnaise
1/2 tbsp crème fraîche
a pinch of sambal oelek

Coarsely chop the shrimp. Core and finely chop the tomato. Mix all the ingredients together and fill up the avocado skin.

1/2 avocado
3 1/2 tbsp (50 g) cottage cheese
3 1/2 tbsp (20 g) sun-dried tomatoes
5 green olives
a pinch of pizza seasoning

Chop the sundried tomatoes and olives. Mix all the ingredients and fill up the avocado skin.

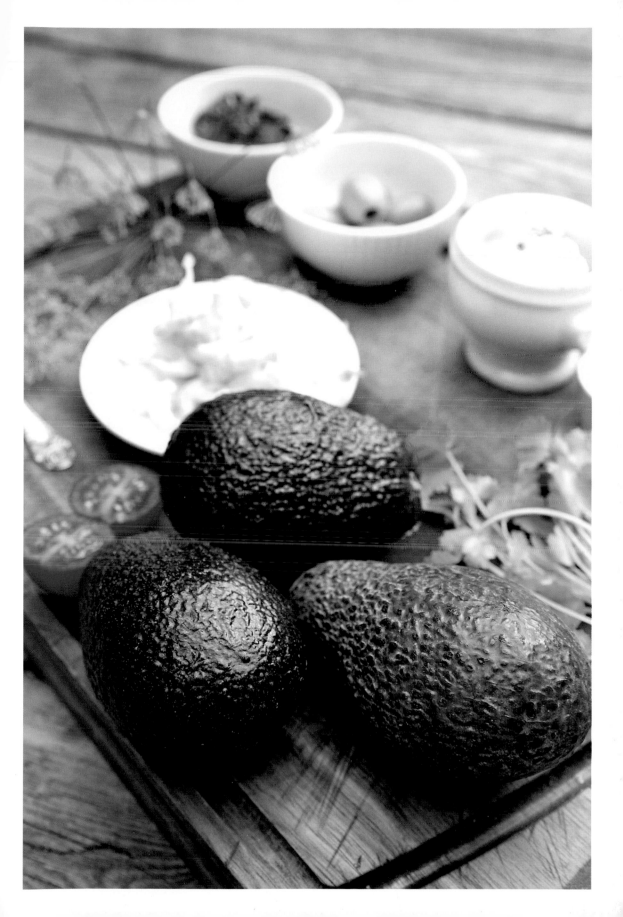

14 SUGGESTIONS FOR LCHQ SNACKS

- Cottage cheese with berries and nuts

- Greek yogurt with berries and nuts

- Plain yogurt with LCHQ granola and berries (see page 60)

- Smoothie with cottage cheese, milk, frozen berries, and ground flaxseed

- Smoothie with Silken tofu, oat milk, frozen berries, and sesame seeds

- Vegetable (e.g. bell peppers, celery, cucumber) and cheese sticks with a couple of olives

- A couple of slices of cooked ham rolled with cheese, peppers, and lettuce

- A mix of plain berries, nuts (e.g. walnuts, pistachio, pumpkin seeds), and dried, unsweetened berries

- A boiled egg and half a grapefruit

- Half an egg with shrimp, a little bit of mayonnaise, and a tomato

- Wild game jerky and approximately 3 1/2 oz (100 g) of honeydew

- A stuffed avocado half (see page 118)

- Strawberry ice cream with chocolate flakes (see page 110)

- A couple of blueberry beads (see page 106)

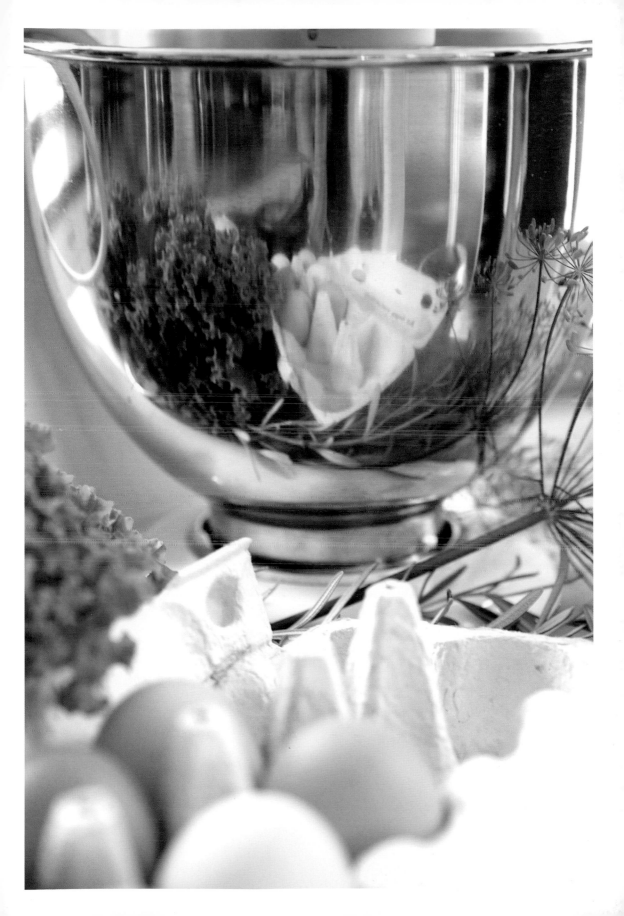

A WEEK
OF LCHQ MEALS

Ⓠ DAY 1
Breakfast: LCHQ granola with plain yogurt and raspberries
Lunch: Summer salad with mackerel, egg, and peas
Dinner: Hot chicken drumsticks with coleslaw

Ⓠ DAY 2
Breakfast: Blueberry smoothie
Lunch: Hot tuna omelet
Dinner: LCHQ mix

Ⓠ DAY 3
Breakfast: Strawberry and coconut smoothie
Lunch: Tofu stir fry
Dinner: Golden cabbage pudding

Ⓠ DAY 4
Breakfast: Breakfast omelet
Lunch: Pickled salmon with a warmed scallion salad
Dinner: Stuffed peppers and portobello mushrooms

Ⓠ DAY 5
Breakfast: LCHQ granola with plain yogurt with raspberries
Lunch: Lemongrass chicken stir fry with a green salad
Dinner: LCHQ root vegetables with salmon and feta

Ⓠ DAY 6
Breakfast: Blueberry smoothie
Lunch: Meat-stuffed eggplants
Dinner: Grilled shrimp scampi with a green salad and avocado cream

Ⓠ DAY 7
Breakfast: LCHQ granola with plain yogurt and raspberries
Lunch: Fish soup with aioli
Dinner: Lemon chicken with oven-baked vegetables
Dessert: Strawberry ice cream with chocolate flakes

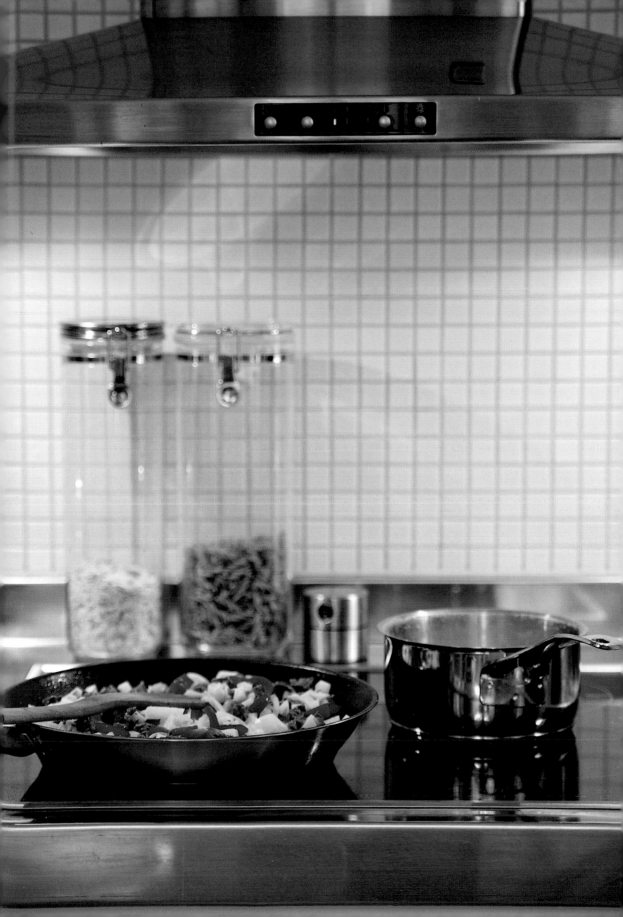

References

1. Perez-Martinez P. et al., Postprandial oxidative stress is modified by dietary fat: evidence from a human intervention study. ClinSci (Lond), Jun 15;119(6):251-61, 2010

2. Fung T.T. et al., Low-Carbohydrate Diets and All-Cause and Cause-Specific Mortality, Annals of Internal Medicine, 153:289-298, 2010

3. Astrup A. et al., The role of reducing intakes of saturated fat in the prevention of cardiovascular disease: where does the evidence stand in 2010? Am. J. Clin. Nutr., Jan 26, 2011

4. Hu F.B., Stampfer M.J., Nut consumption and risk of coronary heart disease: a review of epidemiologic evidence, Current Atherosclerosis Reports 1 (3):204–209, 1999

5. Boyd N.F. et al., Dietary fat and breast cancer risk revisited: a meta-analysis of the published literature, British Journal of Cancer 62 (9):1672–1685, 2003

6. Gonzalez C.A., Riboli E., Diet and cancer prevention: Contributions from the European Prospective Investigation into Cancer and Nutrition (EPIC) study, Eur. J. Cancer Sep;46(14):2555-62, 2010

7. Huncharek M., Kupelnick B., Dietary fat intake and risk of epithelial ovarian cancer: a meta-analysis of 6,689 subjects from 8 observational studies, Nutr. Cancer 40(2):87-91, 2001

8. Alexander D.D. et al, The non-Hodgkin lymphomas: a review of the epidemiologic literature, Int. J. Cancer 120 Suppl. 12:1-39, 2007

9. Cassady B.A. et al., Effects of low carbohydrate diets high in red meats or poultry, fish and shellfish on plasma lipids and weight loss, Nutr. Metab. (Lond) Oct 31;4:23, 2007

10. Arya F. et al., Differences in postprandial inflammatory responses to a 'modern' v. traditional meat meal: a preliminary study, Br. J. Nutr. Sep;104(5):724-8, 2010

11. Mann N., Dietary lean red meat and human evolution, Eur. J. Nutr. Apr;39(2):71-9, 2000

12. Lamont K.T. et al., Is red wine a SAFE sip away from cardioprotection? Mechanisms involved in resveratrol- and melatonin-induced cardioprotection, J. Pineal Res. Feb 23, 2011

13. Yin J. et al., Beverage-specific alcohol intake and bone loss in older men and women: a longitudinal study, Eur. J. ClinNutr. Feb, 2011

14. Natella F. et al., Red wine prevents the postprandial increase in plasma cholesterol oxidation products: a pilot study, Br. J. Nutr. Feb 4:1-6, 2011

15. Andreatta M.M., Dietary patterns and food groups are linked to the risk of urinary tract tumors in Argentina, Eur. J. Cancer Prev. Nov;19(6):478-84, 2010

16. Wong R.H., Acute resveratrol supplementation improves flow-mediated dilatation in overweight/obese individuals with mildly elevated blood pressure, Nutr. Metab. Cardiovasc. Dis. Jul 29, 2010

17. Kalantari H., Das D.K., Physiological effects of resveratrol, Biofactors Sep;36(5):401-6, 2010

18. Yancy W.S. Jr et al., Acid-base analysis of individuals following two weight loss diets, Eur. J. Clin. Nutr. Dec;61(12):1416-22, 2007

19. Dawson-Hughes B., Harris S.S., Ceglia L., Alkaline diets favor lean tissue mass in older adults, Am. J. ClinNutr 87:662-5, 2008

20. McClernon F.J. et al, The effects of a low-carbohydrate ketogenic diet and a low-fat diet on mood, hunger, and other self-reported symptoms, Obesity (Silver Spring) Jan;15(1):182-7, 2007

21. Hahn T.J. et al, Disordered mineral metabolism produced by ketogenic diet therapy, Calcif Tissue Int. Aug 24;28(1):17-22, 1979

22. Gissel T., Poulsen C.S., Vestergaard P., Adverse effects of antiepileptic drugs on bone mineral density in children, Expert Opin. Drug Saf. May;6(3):267-78, 2007

23. Bertoli S. et al, Nutritional status and bone mineral mass in children treated with ketogenic diet, RecentiProg. Med. Dec;93(12):671-5, 2002

24. Johnston C.S. et al, Ketogenic low-carbohydrate diets have no metabolic advantage over nonketogenic low-carbohydrate diets, Am. J. Clin. Nutr. May;83(5):1055-61, 2006

25. Tajalizadekhoob Y. et al, The effect of low-dose omega 3 fatty acids on the treatment of mild to moderate depression in the elderly: a double-blind, randomized, placebo-controlled study, Eur. Arch. Psychiatry Clin. Neurosci., 2011

26. White A.M. et al, Blood ketones are directly related to fatigue and perceived effort during exercise in overweight adults adhering to low-carbohydrate diets for weight loss: a pilot study, J. Am. Diet. Assoc. Oct;107(10):1792-6, 2007

27. Ryan L., Petit S., Addition of whole, semiskimmed, and skimmed bovine milk reduces the total antioxidant capacity of black tea, Nutr. Res. Jan;30(1):14-20, 2010

28. Magrone T., Jirillo E., Polyphenols from red wine are potent modulators of innate and adaptive immune responsiveness, Proc. Nutr. Soc. Aug;69(3):279-85, 2010

29. Hager A. et al., Processing and storage effects on monomeric anthocyanins, percent polymeric color, and antioxidant capacity of processed black raspberry products, J. Food Sci. Aug;73(6):H134-40, 2008

30. Jiménez-Monreal A.M. et al., Influence of cooking methods on antioxidant activity of vegetables, J. Food Sci. Apr;74(3):H97-H103, 2009

31. Cao J.J., Nielsen F.H., Acid diet (high-meat protein) effects on calcium metabolism and bone health, Curr. Opin. Clin. Nutr. Metab. Care. Nov;13(6):698-702, 2010

32. Weigle D.S., A high-protein diet induces sustained reductions in appetite, ad libitum caloric intake, and body weight despite compensatory changes in diurnal plasma leptin and ghrelin concentrations, Am. J. Clin. Nutr. Jul;82(1):41-8, 2005

33. Assunção M.L., Effects of dietary coconut oil on the biochemical and anthropometric profiles of women presenting abdominal obesity, Lipids Jul;44(7):593-601, 2009

34. Portillo M.P., Energy restriction with high-fat diet enriched with coconut oil gives higher UCP1 and lower white fat

in rats, Int. J. Obes. Relat. Metab. Disord. Oct;22(10):974-9, 1998

35. Papamandjaris A.A., Endogenous fat oxidation during medium chain versus long chain triglyceride feeding in healthy women, Int. J. Obes. Relat. Metab. Disord. Sep;24(9):1158-66, 2000

36. St-Onge M.P., Medium- versus long-chain triglycerides for 27 days increases fat oxidation and energy expenditure without resulting in changes in body composition in overweight women, Int. J. Obes. Relat. Metab. Disord. Jan;27(1):95-102, 2003

37. Tsuji H. et al., Dietary medium-chain triacylglycerols suppress accumulation of body fat in a double-blind, controlled trial in healthy men and women, J. Nutr. Nov;131(11):2853-9, 2001

38. Han J.R. et al., Effects of dietary medium-chain triglyceride on weight loss and insulin sensitivity in a group of moderately overweight free-living type 2 diabetic Chinese subjects, Metabolism Jul;56(7):985-91, 2007

39. St-Onge M.P., Jones P.J., Greater rise in fat oxidation with medium-chain triglyceride consumption relative to long-chain triglyceride is associated with lower initial body weight and greater loss of subcutaneous adipose tissue, Int. J. Obes. Relat. Metab. Disord. Dec;27(12):1565-71, 2003

40. St-Onge M.P., Bosarge A., Weight-loss diet that includes consumption of medium-chain triacylglycerol oil leads to a greater rate of weight and fat mass loss than does olive oil, Am. J. Clin. Nutr. Mar;87(3):621-6, 2008

41. St-Onge M.P. et al., Medium-chain triglycerides increase energy expenditure and decrease adiposity in overweight men, Obes. Res. Mar;11(3):395-402, 2003

42. Ogawa A. et al., Dietary medium- and long-chain triacylglycerols accelerate diet-induced thermogenesis in humans, J. Oleo. Sci.56(6):283-7, 2007

43. Pedersen B.K. et al., Role of myokines in exercise and metabolism, J. Appl. Physiol. Sep;103(3):1093-8, 2007

44. Pedersen B.K., Muscles and their myokines, J. Exp. Biol. Jan 15;214(Pt 2):337-46, 2011

45. Watzl B., Anti-inflammatory effects of plant-based foods and of their constituents, Int. J. Vitam. Nutr. Res., Dec;78(6):293-8, 2008

46. Cameron J. et al., A high-fat diet impairs cardiac high-energy phosphate metabolism and cognitive function in healthy human subjects, Am. J. Clin. Nutr. 93:748-755, 2011

47. de Koning L. et al., Low-carbohydrate diet scores and risk of type 2 diabetes in men, Am. J. Clin. Nutr. Vol 93 No 4; 844-850, 2011

48. Hamilton-Reeves J.M. et al., Clinical studies show no effects of soy protein or isoflavones on reproductive hormones in men: results of a meta-analysis, Fertil. Steril. Aug;94(3):997-1007, 2010

49. O'Neil C.E. et al., Relationship between 100 procent juice consumption and nutrient intake and weight of adolescents, Am. J. Health Promot. Mar-Apr;24(4):231-7, 2010

50. Schroder K.E., Effects of fruit consumption on body mass index and weight loss in a sample of overweight and obese dieters enrolled in a weight-loss intervention trial, Nutrition Dec 17, 2009

51. Alinia S., Hels O., Tetens I., The potential association between fruit intake and body weight – a review, Obes. Rev. Nov;10(6):639-47, 2009

52. Kianbakht S., Ghazavi A., Immunomodulatory Effects of Saffron: A Randomized Double-Blind Placebo-Controlled Clinical Trial, Phytother. Res. Apr 8. doi: 10.1002/ptr.3484, 2011

53. Kulkarni S.K., Bhutani M.K., Bishnoi M., Antidepressant activity of curcumin: involvement of serotonin and dopamine system, Psychopharmacology (Berl) Dec;201(3):435-42, 2008

54. Mao Q.Q. et al., Involvement of serotonergic system in the antidepressant-like effect of piperine, Prog. Neuropsychopharmacol Biol. Psychiatry, Apr 6, 2011

55. Bhattacharya A. et al, Allylisothiocyanate-rich mustard seed powder inhibits bladder cancer growth and muscle invasion, Carcinogenesis Dec;31(12):2105-10, 2010

56. Butt M.S., Sultan M.T., Ginger and its 'health claims: molecular aspects, Crit. Rev. Food Sci. Nutr. May;51(5):383-93, 2011

57. Yamaguchi M., Regulatory mechanism of food factors in bone metabolism and prevention of osteoporosis, Yakugaku Zasshi Nov;126(11):1117-37, 2006

58. Davis P.A., Yokoyama W., Cinnamon Intake Lowers Fasting Blood Glucose: Meta-Analysis, J. Med. Food Apr 11, 2011

59. Ng T.P. et al., Curry consumption and cognitive function in the elderly, Am. J. Epidemiol. Nov 1;164(9):898-906, 2006

60. Chandrasekara N., Shahidi F., Effect of Roasting on Phenolic Content and Antioxidant Activities of Whole Cashew Nuts, Kernels, and Testa, J. Agric. Food Chem. Mar 25, 2011

61. Damasceno N.R. et al., Crossover study of diets enriched with virgin olive oil, walnuts or almonds. Effects on lipids and other cardiovascular risk markers, Nutr. Metab. Cardiovasc. Dis. Mar 21, 2011

62. Thomson C.D. et al., Brazil nuts: an effective way to improve selenium status, Am. J. Clin. Nutr. Feb;87(2):379-84, 2008

63. Lucas L., Russell A., Keast R., Molecular mechanisms of inflammation. Anti-inflammatory benefits of virgin olive oil and the phenolic compound oleocanthal, Curr. Pharm. Des. 17(8):754-68, 2011

64. Waterman E., Lockwood B., Active components and clinical applications of olive oil, Altern. Med. Rev. Dec;12(4):331-42, 2007

65. Iggman D. et al., Replacing dairy fat with rapeseed oil causes rapid improvement of hyperlipidaemia: a randomised controlled study, J. Intern. Med. Apr 5, 2011

66. Hooper L. et al., Reduced or modified dietary fat for preventing cardiovascular disease, Cochrane Database Syst. Rev. Jul 6;(7):CD002137, 2011

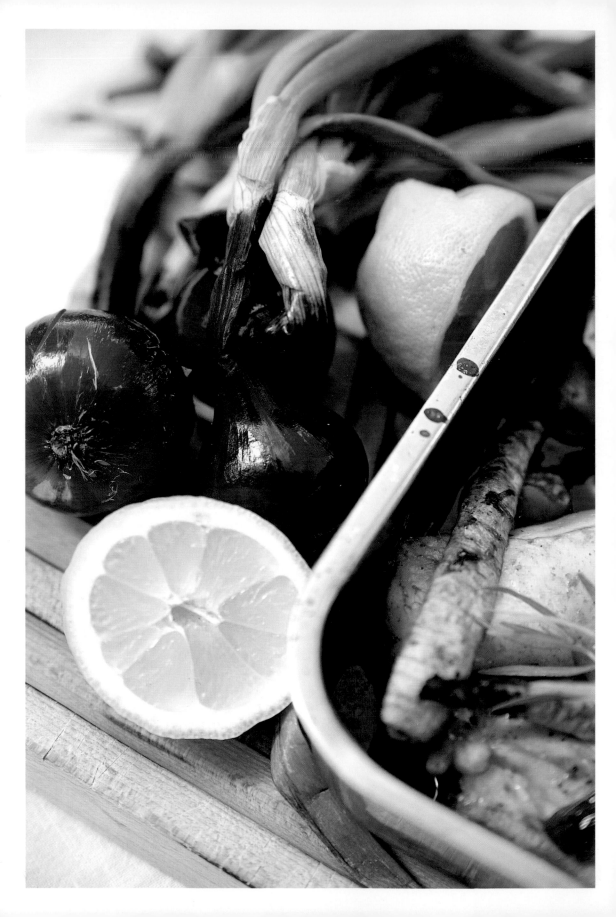

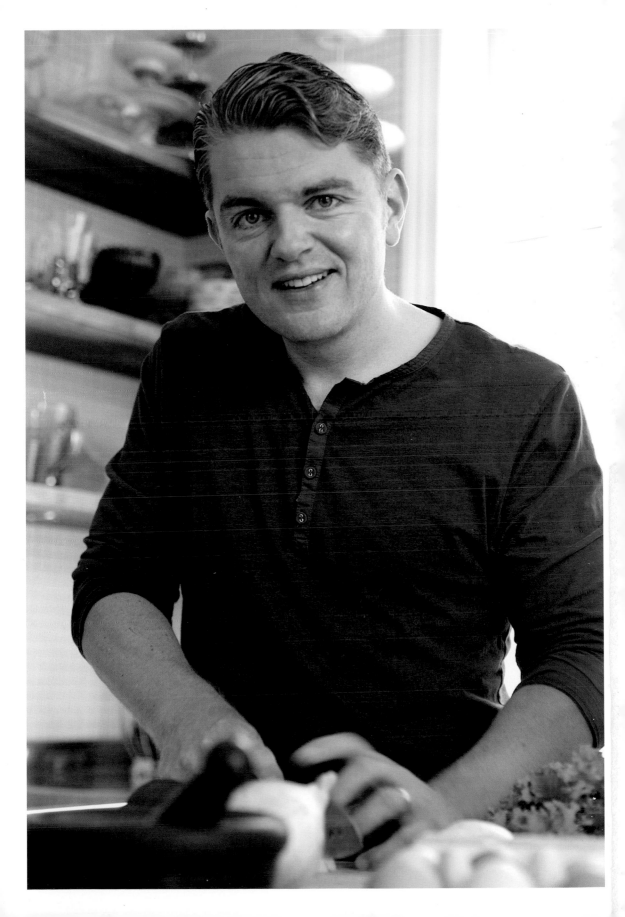

Recipe Index

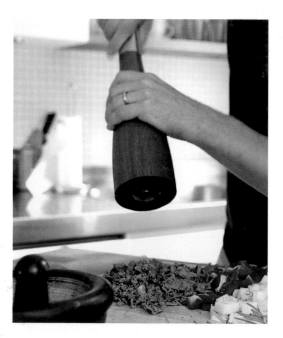